Registered with the FDA and patented by the Korea Intellectual Property Office

CBK Splint

Cranial Balancing Key Splint

Improves Your Whole-body Health

Byungkee Choi & Youngkyun Choi

Well 도서출판 웰

도서출판 웰

01041. 22, Samyang-ro 118 gil, Gangbuk-gu, Seoul, Korea
T. 82. 2. 907. 2872 F. 82. 2. 907. 2873
E. bkc905@hanmail.net
H. www.wellpub.net

This book was originally pubished in Korea
under the title of :

CBK Splint **Improves Your Whole-body Health**

ISBN. 978-89-97113-79-8 93510

Printed in Korea

Testimonials 1

Kung-Rock Kwon

- President of Korean Academy of Dental Science,
- Professor of Kyung Hee University School of Dentistry

My relationship with Director Byungkee Choi, who is now deceased, goes back over 20 years. We met for the first time as new directors of the Korean Academy of Stomatognathic Function and occlusion when we were young, and since then we have not only had academic exchanges, but have also worked together in various fields of the dental field, giving each other help and forming a friendship. Although the author was in private practice as a dentist, he did not neglect academic research. In particular, he studied occlusion, a field that others avoid, continuously and persistently, and achieved good results through many clinical trials. Seeing him publish the results of his diligent research in a book makes me respect and envy him. And as a public official myself, I write a letter of recommendation carefully while feeling guilty about my laziness toward academics.

In dental clinical practice, occlusion is a very important and fundamental area of treatment, so it is a field that cannot be overemphasized, and the theories are diverse. Now, while many fields of dental science have established theoretical foundations and applied them to clinical practice to ensure predictable treatment results, in the field of occlusion, various theories and clinical applications still coexist.

The author has developed his own treatment method and applied it to patients in order to find evidence for a stable prognosis while treating patients. He also organized extensive clinical data over a long period of time and presented it to dental clinicians through lectures and in print. I applaud the author's academic passion and persistence in completing this book.

In this book, the author explains the application of occlusal treatment using 'CBK (Cranial Balancing Key) Splint' and its effects. On the one hand, there is some overemphasis on the effects of splints, but it is already widely known that there is a close relationship between overall health and occlusal balance.

In particular, in order to prove the effectiveness of treatment, the author not only presented an objective and standardized application method using an occlusal measurement device called T-Scan on various patients with occlusal problems, and objectively investigated the results. Its characteristic feature is that it also collects the patient's subjective treatment experience.

Through this book, the author emphasizes the importance of occlusal treatment. It can be seen that the author has tried to help not only professional clinicians but also the general public understand dental occlusion by organizing the contents of occlusion in various medical fields through 30 years of clinical experience.

Through this book, the author is trying his best to provide evidence for his techniques and experiences regarding occlusion, and, more importantly, to talk about the life and service of a dentist. All judgment on this remains the responsibility of all of us who read this book.

I miss Director Byungkee Choi even more at this time today.

2023. 9.

After listening to the 'CBK Splint' lectured by Byungkee Choi (16th President of I.C.D Korea)

Yang Shok Yoo (former Physician to the President)

I was truly moved by Dr. Byungkee Choi's excellent lecture titled "Correlation between occlusion and periodontal disease and correlation between systemic disease and CBK (cranial balancing key) Splint."

I was even more impressed by the development and expansion of the dental field in terms of its correlation with systemic diseases. I believe that this is a challenge that the entire dental community must solve, and that it is a task that needs to be studied globally.

As someone who has personally experienced the 70-year history of the development of Korean dental medicine, I believe that Dr. Choi's lecture is an issue that must be explored as epoch-making new scholarship.

While serving in the military, I achieved rapid progress in dentistry, especially maxillofacial oral surgery, amidst conflict with general military doctors (M.Cs).

Dentistry has not only oral surgery but also oral medicine. As someone who emphasizes the relationship between dentistry and systemic diseases, I was proud and envious of Dr. Choi's research and achievements.

I have experienced losing my maxillary premolar and molar teeth due to Traumatic Occlusion. So I listened to this lecture more carefully than anyone else and thought I should wear the CBK Splint.

I mourn Dr. Choi, who passed away at such a young age, and hope that he rests in peace in heaven.

Foreword

My father, Dr. Byungkee Choi, has been curious about the efficacy of splints since he was attending dental school a long time ago. One day, while practicing as a dentist, he noticed that a patient suffering from temporomandibular joint pain showed improvement in his overall health after receiving splint treatment, and began researching the effects of splints.

My father searched for the answer to this question while studying dental occlusion. He learned that occlusion is generally related to dental health by having a great impact on periodontal tissue, but that a good occlusion also has a positive effect on whole-body health.

While he was a board member of Korean Academy of Stomatognathic Function and Occlusion, he conducted research on occlusal theory with many professors. He exchanged with Dr. R.B. Kerstein in the United States about the clinical concept of occlusal adjustment using T-scan, and created a therapeutic philosophy for occlusion.

My father presented the correlation between occlusion and periodontal disease at the Korean Association of Temporo-Occlusion in 2009. He introduced in a textbook on temporomandibular joint occlusion that occlusal abnormalities can have a worse impact on periodontal disease than plaque. The main content was that occlusal adjustment using T-scan and the splint that complements it play an important role in the health and preservation of periodontal tissue.

Afterwards, through continued research and accumulated data, he saw the possibility that splints could improve whole-body health, and he studied the relationship between the temporomandibular joint, occlusion, and whole-body health for several years to solve the original riddle he had as an undergraduate. My father, who studied occlusion, paid attention to the relationship between temporomandibular joint distortion and overall health, like the previous research by Mark. A. Piper and P. Dawson, believed that dental occlusion was the cause and explored this field further.

In September 2015, he presented "Cranial Balancing Key (CBK) Splint and Anti-aging Effects" at the 16th International College of Prosthodontists (ICP) Conference. Professor Heo SeongJoo, Professor Kung-Rock Kwon, and Dental hospital director Colonel Dong Soo Park(8th United States Army, EUSA) helped him a lot.

In the presentation at the time, my father said that he performs occlusal adjustments to match the centric relation of the teeth with maximal intercuspation. It was said that the deficiencies after bite adjustment can be compensated by wearing a CBK Splint when sleeping or exercising. As a result, it was introduced that it has the potential to improve periodontal disease, improve sleep quality, rhinitis, tinnitus, facial shape, and increase blood flow to the brain, and was greatly approved by the attendees.

My father worked with doctors in other departments to study the good effects seen in over 5,000 cases at his hospital. And he tried to contribute to human health by making this known to the world.

One of the important contents included in the CBK Splint concept is '5 Components of Whole-Body Health'. These are: 1) Straighten your back with proper posture, 2) Use the CBK Splint well, 3) Do abdominal breathing, 4) Meditate, 5) Well diet and Exercise. Along with how to use the Splint, My father educate his patients about 5 Components of Whole -Body Health and get good effects. I would like to express my sincere gratitude to the patients of our clinic who have actively followed my father's theory.

I also did my residency and Ph.D. in Prosthodontics at Kyung-Hee University School of Dentistry, where I was able to learn about the theory of occlusion and the importance of occlusion. I would like to thank all the professors from the Department of Prosthodontics at Kyung-Hee University including Professor Kung-Rock Kwon for teaching me this. And I am especially grateful to my father, who taught me directly from the sidelines.

When my father passed away suddenly on Monday, February 27, 2023, I was unable to do anything for a while because the vacancy he left behind was too big. A few months later, when I came to my senses, I thought, 'I need to publicize my father's achievements as a dentist to the world and leave his name in history.' As my first activity since my father's death, I participated in 'The 8th International Invention Innovation Competition in Canada' in Toronto, Canada in August 2023 with the concept of CBK Splint and won the prize. Then I collected the manuscripts my father had left unfinished and published them as the book "CBK Splint." I decided to introduce the concept of CBK Splint by distributing this book to foreign dentists attending the International College of Dentists (ICD) convention held in Korea in November 2023. I am also preparing several papers on CBK Splint.

My father always like to care for patients in need and provided medical services to local schools and churches. Even during his summer vacation, he used to go to Mongolia, Thailand, and the Philippines to provide medical service instead of going to a summer resort. When I was in middle school, I followed my father to Mongolia and participated in medical volunteer service. As I watched my father go to remote areas of Mongolia where there were no medical facilities and serve the local people devotedly, I began to dream of becoming a dentist when I grew up.

Here's what my father always told me.

"I want to improve the health of people around the world with CBK Splint"

I have always kept these words in my heart and honored the will of my father. I will continue to do so with that as my mission.

Lastly, I would like to express my gratitude to Professor Kung-Rock Kwon(Kyung-hee university School of Dentistry), Advisor Yang Shok Yoo (former physician to the president), Professor Jae Hyun Park(Arizona School of Dentistry & Oral Health), Principal Bongki Cheon, Professor Chidong Kim(Seoul National University of Science and Technology), Director Dong soo Park(Former 8th US Army(Yongsan) Dental hospital director), Manager Eunhye Lee and our hospital staffs who helped me pubilsh my father's posthumous work. And I would like to express my sincere gratitude to my mother, Hyunsook Son, who devotedly helped my father achieve such achievements. I would also like to thank my wife Kyoungsun Lim, my sister Min-Hee Choi, her husband Byung-Kwan Kim, grandson Jinyul Choi and granddaughter Chae-Ahn Kim who always supported me by my father's side.

Foreword

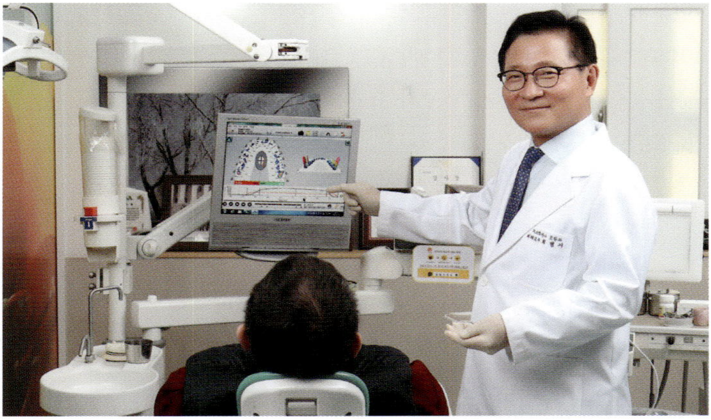

My father in Heaven!

My father worked all his life and then went to heaven. Please always watch over me from heaven. Sometimes you come to me in my dreams and guide me on the way. I will do my best. I respect and love you with all my heart. Rest in peace.

November 3rd, 2023

Posted by son Youngkyun Choi

Contents

chapter 03 Dental Clinical Effects of CBK Splints

chapter 04 CBK Splints and Whole-body Health

chapter 01

What is a 'CBK Splint' ?

01 The concept of and motivation for 'CBK Splints'

02 Basic concept and characteristics of the CBK Splint

03 Clinical effects of wearing a CBK Splint

04 CBK Splints and Whole-body Health

05 Future development prospects of CBK Splint

01 The concept of and motivation for 'CBK Splints'

In the past, it was thought that periodontal disease (tooth loss) was caused by not brushing teeth well enough. The theory has changed somewhat recently and the mainstream thinking now is that periodontal disease is often caused by an abnormality in occlusion. This is because when teeth mesh with incorrect occlusion, they are subject to a lot of force on one side, causing distortion of the masticatory muscles. This leads to further misalignment of the teeth, which in turn continues to adversely affect the gums, and has an even greater impact on gum disease.

I fully discuss these issues in Textbook of human jaw function & occlusion which wrote in 2014. Since then, I have continued to research the effects malocclusions on the health of the whole body.

When an occlusion is misaligned, not just the masticatory muscles are distorted, but the skull can be distorted, too, and the brain and spinal cord are also affected. In other words, as the teeth become worn and twisted, the skull is affected as well, and this affects the immune system and health of the entire body.

To solve these problems, the CBK Splint (cranial balancing key) was created.

02 Basic concept and characteristics of the CBK Splint

The CBK splint is an individualized occlusal splint, optimized according to each patient's dental structure. It is fabricated using a metal strip bite which allows the occlusion to be positioned in a centric relation, and provides 1.5 ㎜ of space in the posterior teeth that have been adjusted for proper occlusion.

What makes CBK Splints different from other splints?

First, after checking the occlusion of a patient's teeth using a T-scan and adjusting it to the ideal occlusion, a splint bite is fabricated. In this way, it has structural features optimized for each patient.

Second, the core technology of splint production lies in the thickness of the metal strip bite. When a patient is in the most comfortable state, about 1.5~2 ㎜ of space is created in the posterior teeth. If the space between upper and lower posterior teeth is greater than 1.5~2 ㎜, too much tensile force will act on the temporomandibular joint, potentially causing discomfort and temporomandibular joint disorders. If it is less than 1.5~2 ㎜, the device could break, reducing the effectiveness of the splint.

Therefore, it is most desirable when the optimum thickness of the splint is 1.5~2 ㎜. Through some trial and error and several experiments, I succeeded in making a metal strip bite with a thickness of 1.5~2 ㎜ by taking three 0.7 ㎜ perforated aluminum metal strips (0.4~0.5 ㎜ thick) inside the bite and overlapped them to form a 1.5~2 ㎜ thick metal strip bite which has been recognized as a creative invention technology and was given a patent by the Korean Intellectual Property Office.

Third, it was developed to improve the health of the whole body, expanding the concept of dental health within the oral cavity to encompass whole-body health. Occlusion and temporomandibular joint abnormalities directly affect the cervical spine and skull. The CBK Splint improves overall whole-body health by stabilizing the endocrine system (hormones) and nervous systems by stabilizing the occlusion and temporomandibular joint.

03 Clinical effects of wearing a CBK Splint

In order to maintain healthy teeth, it is necessary to maintain optimal occlusion. It has been known for some time that periodontal disease can be caused by improper brushing of the teeth, but an even greater negative effect is caused by poor occlusion. In other words, many diseases such as periodontal disease, cervical abrasion, and cracked teeth can occur due to occlusal interference. This is especially true at night when some people grind and clench their teeth, and may swallow saliva as often as once a minute. In severe cases, occlusal forces 6~10 times greater than normal direct a destructive force to the teeth. The tooth destruction due to occlusal forces is worst when people are unconscious while they sleep. Fortunately, occlusal interference is eliminated when CBK Splints are worn. They have the effect of removing the destructive force of the masticatory muscles that occurs during sleep when the occlusion is not correct. And they reduce the occlusal force to create an appropriate periodontal condition.

What are the benefits of CBK splints in clinical treatment?

First, when the occlusal force of the teeth stops acting destructively, the teeth or gingiva no longer deteriorate.

When CBK Splints are worn while sleeping, they relieve the occlusion force and thus play an important role in relieving periodontal or occlusion disease. Therefore, people with periodontal disease should wear a CBK Splint.

Second, CBK splints promote a deeper sleep.

During sleep, people perform swallowing exercises that activate the brain by stimulating it once a minute. When this happens, adults with occlusal disease with severe tooth wear can receive 6~10 times more than the normal occlusal force, which is a major cause of not being able to sleep deeply. The CBK splint relieves the force even when swallowing, leading to a much more comfortable sleep.

Third, CBK Splints promote hormonal balance and the nervous system function, thus helping to promote the whole-body health.

CBK Splints can help people to recover from systemic diseases such as rhinitis, tinnitus, and migraine.

When a CBK Splint is worn, the traction force that increases the cervical 1st (atlas) and cervical 2nd (axis) vertebrae helps to correct alignment of the spine. As a result, the abnormal symptoms of the cranial nerves and cerebrospinal fluid caused by the fine twisting of the cervical vertebrae 1 and 2 are restored. If an occlusion does not fit well, the teeth wear and the cervical vertebrae become distorted. In particular, the temporomandibular joint affects 272 muscles (136 muscles each side). Therefore, malocclusion of the teeth directly affects the temporomandibular joints and spine. When the spine is distorted, blood pressure rises, tinnitus occurs, and many incurable diseases such as rhinitis can develop.

Proper posture and wearing a CBK Splint promote normalization of hormones and the nervous system and increase immunity. When the spine is upright, all immune cells, that is, T cells, B cells, and NK cells, can respond immediately. Twisting of the cervical vertebrae and pelvis caused by dental occlusion abnormalities along with bad posture causes the spine to bend. Therefore, proper posture and dental occlusion stabilization are essential conditions for whole-body health.

Fourth, facial asymmetry is alleviated, and the face becomes beautiful through a balance of hormones caused by the stabilization of the pituitary gland.

If there is occlusal interference, the muscular distortion and twisting are 7~8 times greater in the masticatory muscles and the medial and lateral pterygoid muscles. As a result, the twenty-two sphenoid and temporal bones which constitute the most central part of the skull become twisted.

Most of the cranial nerves emerge from the sphenoid bone, and hormones are produced by the pituitary gland above the sphenoid bone. As we age, teeth wear out which has an effect on the sphenoid bone, resulting in facial asymmetry, that is, distortion of the eyes and nose. Therefore, wearing a CBK Splint corrects facial asymmetry to some extent and restores the face to its correct shape. In addition, the CBK Splint helps to smooth the movement of hormones and cerebrospinal fluid which improves health in general.

Fifth, CBK Splints can help to prevent dementia by increasing blood flow to the brain.

As the average lifespan of humans increases, the elderly population also increases and there is a corresponding increase in the number of people with dementia. It is known that 60~70 % of dementia patients have symptoms caused by Alzheimer's disease. By the way, Alzheimer's disease is a neurological condition in which brain nerve cells gradually die as amyloid beta-42 protein decreases in the brain tissue while tau protein increases and accumulates in the brain. Therefore, since dental occlusion affects the flow of the skull and pituitary fluid, CBK splints that correct occlusion can be a way to reduce the likelihood of developing dementia.

Sixth, CBK Splints can slow facial aging caused by distortion of the spine and skull due to destructive occlusion forces.

If the force applied to the muscles is ideally minimized to 12 ㎏/㎠ by aligning the centric relation and maximal intercuspal position with a CBK Splint, the force applied to the facial muscles can be adjusted to affect the nasolabial folds and shape of the face.

To summarize the effects of wearing a CBK Splint,

(1) Normal temporomandibular joint disk space is secured.

(2) The traction force of the upper cervical vertebrae loosens the knotted muscles in the neck.

(3) It affects the stabilization of cranial movement.

(4) By removing occlusal interference, it has the effect of preventing 6~10 times more destructive force from reaching the masticatory muscles during sleep when the occlusion is not correct.

(5) The imbalance between the temporal bone and the occipital bone is eliminated.

In more than 5,000 cases in which CBK Splints were worn, I have been able to witness many good results such as a reduction of periodontal disease, tinnitus, rhinitis, and nasolabial folds, accompanied by an improvement in immunity, facial features, and sleep quality.

04 CBK Splints and Whole-body Health

I introduced the 'Five Components of Whole-body Health' during the presentation of a thesis on 'CBK (Cranial Balancing Key) Splints & Anti-Aging Effects' at the 16th International College of Prosthodontists (ICP) in 2015.

The Five Components of Whole-body Health are:

One - Correct spine posture.

This is the most important component. As Gerald. H. Smith announced, "Diseases are induced in the human body as the skull, temporomandibular joints, pelvis, nutrition, muscles, organs, and mental problems mutually and organically interact with each other. Each organ is connected to one of the 24 vertebrae. If posture is incorrect, organ functions can be reduced by 20~30 %.

Keeping the spine upright stabilizes the nervous system and endocrine (hormones) that are affected by the skull and spine which improves overall health.

Two – Correct occlusion of the teeth.

If the dental occlusion is not correct or is distorted, the four masticatory (chewing) muscles can be distorted by 6~10 times more than in ideal cases. This distorts the temporal bone and the second cervical vertebrae (axial vertebrae), which are the most important bones in the human body. This phenomenon mainly happens when people swallow while in an unconscious state during sleep. At that time, occlusal diseases such as cervical abrasion, articulation, cracked teeth, and tooth mobility are induced. A T-scan can be used to check for occlusal disease so the teeth can be adjusted to an ideal occlusion like that of a young person. If this is not enough, a CBK Splint made of a 1.5 ㎜ metal strip bite should be worn during sleep and while exercising. In this way, the lower part of the medial pterygoid muscle will be completely relaxed, ultimately minimizing the influence of muscle distortion on the skull by balancing the upper and lower jaws correctly.

Three - Correct abdominal breathing.

Stress is the root of all diseases. Abdominal breathing helps to control the autonomic nerves and boost immunity, thus reducing the risk of disease. You can breathe from your abdomen by relaxing all the muscles in your body, lying comfortably on the floor and closing your eyes. Place one hand on your stomach and the other on your chest so you can feel the muscle movement as you breathe. With the hand that is on your stomach, feel it expand as you slowly and deeply inhale as much as possible through your nose for 2~4 seconds. Keeping your shoulders and chest still, hold your breath for 2~4 seconds. When exhaling, purse your lips and exhale as slowly as possible for about 4~8 seconds, making a whistling sound as you exhale.

Four - Correct mind control.

It has been said that people can achieve whatever they think. It is important to minimize thoughts of the past and future and focus mainly on the present. Meditation can be used as a way to control the mind, but it is effective only when it is preceded by considerable training for some time. Meditation has a positive effect on the autonomic nervous system and the flow of hormones, so it contributes to psychological stability and relieves stress, which is helpful for whole-body health. Possibly the best part of meditation is that it can be done and enjoyed on an individual basis.

Five – Correct environment (Diet and exercise).

Modern people have come to realize the importance of proper diet and exercise. In the past, malnutrition was a problem, but now, overnutrition is the cause of many diseases. Health-conscious people choose uncontaminated, clean foods and eat a balanced intake of nutrients their bodies need.

Exercise should be tailored to the physical strength and

conditioning of each individual. It needs to become a regular habit, so each part of the body can work smoothly.

05 Future development prospects of CBK Splint

In the future, we plan to expand the use and application of CBK Splints through joint research with many other departments such as internal medicine, otolaryngology, neurology, orthopedics, oriental medicine, and secure clinical evidence for various effects. Recently, the number of patients with dementia has been rapidly increasing, and since dementia is related to the flow of pituitary fluid, pituitary fluid testing is being used to diagnose dementia. Since dental occlusion affects the flow of the skull and pituitary fluid, we will continue research to find a correlation between CBK splints that correct occlusion and prevent dementia.

By introducing newly developed cutting-edge manufacturing technologies such as 3D printing, we plan to develop splints that are more precise and suitable for individual tooth structures. If mass production becomes possible through innovation in manufacturing technology, it is expected that the unit cost of splints will be reduced, thus lifting some of the financial burden on patients.

CBK Splints received a patent from the Korean Intellectual Property Office in 2015 as a creative invention named 'Metal Strip Bite.' In 2016, it was registered as a 'Medical Device' by the US

FDA and DOHS (California Department of Health). Based on this technology recognized domestically and internationally, I plan to expand the supply to the world, including the United States and Europe, starting with Japan, China, and Southeast Asia, which have many similarities with Korea.

It is my humble dream to see people around the world wearing CBK Splints every night and enjoying a healthy and happy life. I would be pleased if the splints were as essential to everyone today as the smart phone.

chapter 02

CBK Splints & Anti-aging Effects

01 Overview of the CBK Splint Thesis

1 Thesis title

CBK (CRANIAL BALANCING KEY) SPLINTS & ANTI-AGING EFFECTS

- D.D.S., Ph. D., F.I.C.D., Byungkee Choi / Choi Byungkee Dental Clinic, Seoul, Korea -

2 Thesis presented at the 16th International College of Prosthodontists (ICP) Conference in 2015

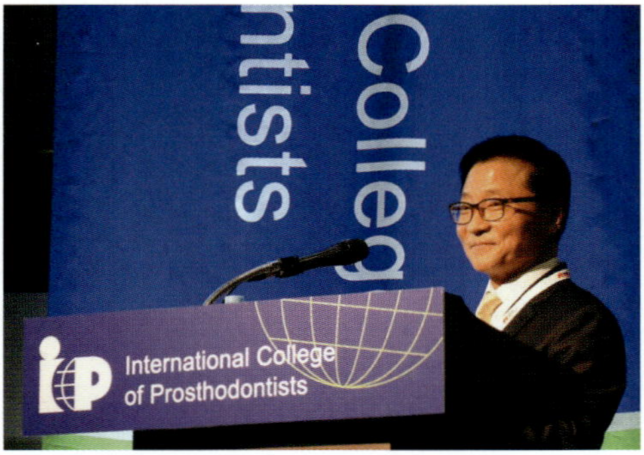

▲ Fig 1. Thesis presentation

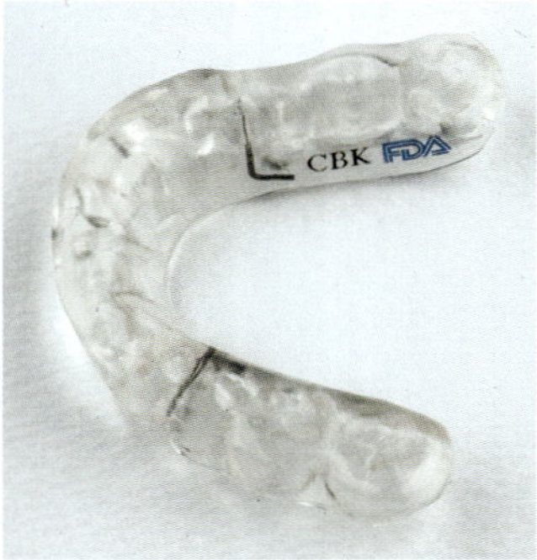

▲ Fig 2. A CBK Splint

The 16th academic conference of the International College of Prosthodontists (ICP), with more than 70 member countries, was held at COEX, Seoul, from September 17 to 20, 2015. At this symposium, about 50 invited speakers gave lectures on about 10 topics such as CAD/CAM, CERAMICS, GERIATRICS, IMPLANTS, MAXILLO-FACIAL, OCCLUSION, and PRACTICE.

More specifically, great lectures were given by world-renowned experts such as Professor John Beumer (USA, Maxillo-Facial field), Professor Rhonda Jacob (USA), Professor Nicola Zitzmann (Switzerland, prosthetic treatment field), and Professor Thomas Taylor (USA, implant field). They drew a lot of attention. Ten of the lecturers were from Korea, and guests from around the world were introduced to the advanced level of Korean prosthetics.

I was honored to be invited to speak at this world-renowned ICP academic conference, lecturing on the topic of 'CBK (Cranial Balancing Key) Splint & Anti-aging Effects.' My lecture on the core part of dental prosthetic treatment was well-received and highly praised by the attendees.

3 Thesis abstract

The CBK (Cranial Balancing Key) Splint is a personalized occlusal device that is manufactured by acquiring precise information about the patient's individual tooth structure. The basic concept is that the CBK Splint creates 1.5~2 ㎜ of space in the occlusally adjusted posterior teeth when the device is worn.

When the CBK Splint is used during sleep or exercise, occlusal stress caused by bruxism or force generated when swallowing can be reduced. In addition, the splint protects teeth from external forces and plays a role in stabilizing the central and peripheral nervous systems through the traction of the atlas (C1) and axis (C2) vertebrae. These effects can reduce tinnitus, rhinitis, and migraines. It is known that nine cranial nerves affect the 'temporo-mandibular joint.'

In particular, the 5th cranial nerve, the trigeminal nerve, is connected to the axis. Most patients with problems in this area are likely to have occlusal diseases such as attrition, flexion fractures, hypersensitivity, and muscle pain.

After adjusting the occlusion using the T-scan III, even if the centric relations slides in a patient wearing a CBK Splint, an ideal occlusion is formed on the Splint, so teeth and surrounding tissues can be protected.

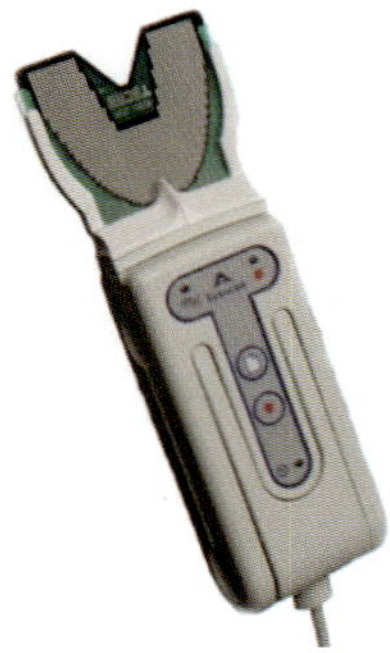

▲ Fig 3. T-scan core handle

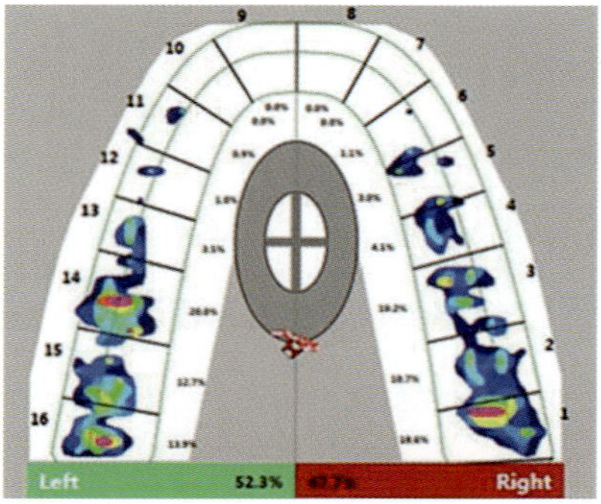

▲ Fig 4. T-scan software view

T-scan is a device that measures occlusal force using a pressure sensor and saves the information as a computer graphic video relative to time. It can reliably detect abnormal teeth meshing down to 0.01 ㎜.

CBK Splints produce several effects when uses for dental treatment:

First, CBK Splints reduce the destructive force generated during sleep through complete relaxation of the inferior belly of the pterygoid muscle. As a result, the occlusal force is reduced, and a desirable periodontal condition is created.

Second, sleep quality can be improved in many patients using CBK Splints. This is thought to be due to a reduction of the abnormally strong occlusal force caused by swallowing, which occurs once a minute during sleep.

Third, CBK Splints distribute the tensile force applied to the temporo-mandibular joint which creates a normal arrangement of the atlas and axis vertebrae. Through these CBK effects, the immune system is activated, which helps maintain the homeostasis of the nervous system.

Fourth, many people have an asymmetrical face. CBK splints can create a symmetrical face by relaxing the fixation of the parieto-temporal and occipito-temporal parts.

Fifth, centric relation is the most important concept in whole-body health. CBK Splints are intended to achieve an ideal occlusion while they balance and stabilize the skull by completely relaxing the inferior belly of the pterygoid muscle.

How to solve occlusion problems

1) Occlusal adjustment

- Using T-scan III, make the Occlusal time within 0.3 seconds and the disclusion time within 0.4 seconds.

2) Cranial Balancing Key (CBK) Splint

- Matches the centric relation and maximal intercuspal position during sleep and exercise.

Conclusion

Unlike conventional splints, the core of the CBK Splint is made of a 1.5 mm-thick metal strip bite, adding a new concept for intraoral treatment that includes occlusal adjustment. More importantly, it extends the concept of occlusion to whole-body health using a CBK Splint and spine erection exercises.

Wearing a CBK Splint helps to improve immunity by stabilizing the spine and skull, which have a decisive effect on the control of the autonomic nervous system. The splints can be one way to slow down the aging process caused by distortion of the spine and skull caused by destructive occlusal forces.

For the health of the whole body, correct spine posture, abdominal breathing, proper diet and exercise, and a positive mindset are necessary.

Healthy stretching with a CBK Splint

< Effect >

- By aligning the 1st and 2nd cervical vertebrae, the passage of foramen magnum between the brain and the trunk remains unhindered.

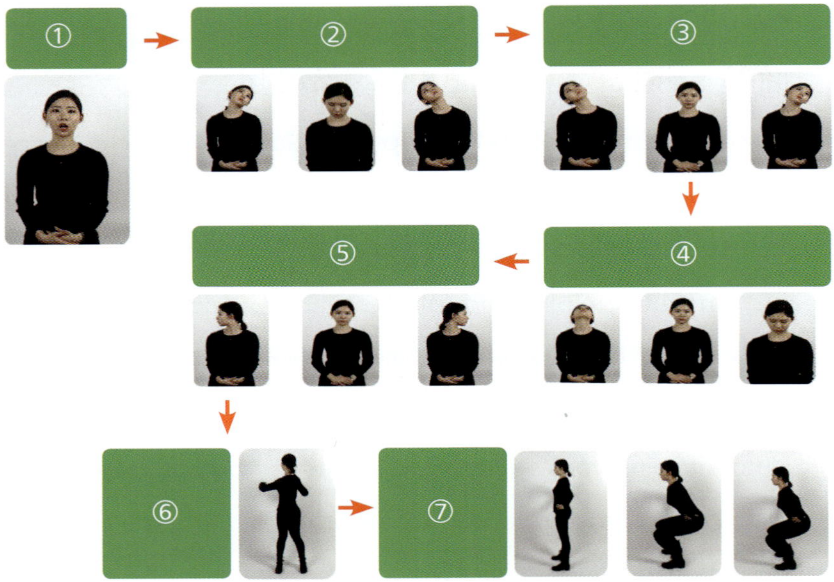

▲ Fig 5. Healthy stretching with a CBK Splint

① Exercises to open and close the jaw

② Left and right neck rotation exercise (neck rotation exercise)

③ Bending the head to the left and right (left and right lateral flexion)

④ Bending the head back and forth (forward and backward flexion)

⑤ Left and right horizontal rotation of the head (horizontal rotation)

⑥ Exercises that relax the body by horizontally rotating and twisting it from side to side

⑦ Exercise in which you sit down and stand up repeatedly in an upright position

02 Principles of the CBK Splint

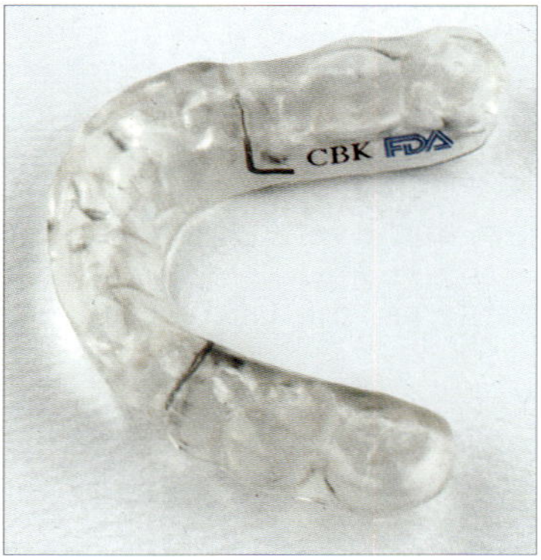

▲ Fig 6. CBK(cranial balancing key) Splint

1 Motivation for the development of CBK Splint

In the past, it was thought that not brushing teeth caused gingiva disease and the need for tooth extraction. However, recently, many teeth are being extracted due to occlusion abnormalities. If the occlusion is not correct when the teeth mesh, considerable force is applied to one side, causing muscle distortion. Therefore, the understanding that most tooth extraction is due to malocclusion has become prevalent. These occlusion abnormalities adversely affect tissues around the teeth and furthermore cause periodontal disease. In 2014, the above information was summarized and published in an occlusal textbook. In addition, the effects of occlusion on whole-body health have been continuously studied. When the occlusion is misaligned, muscle distortion occurs and the skull is distorted, affecting the brain and spinal cord. In other words, it has been recognized that as teeth wear and occlusion deteriorates, this affects the skull, spine, and overall health and immune system.

To solve these problems, the CBK Splint was developed and is being used clinically.

2 Basic concept of the CBK Splint

A CBK Splint is a type of centric relation splint, similar in shape to the mouthpiece worn by boxers and other athletes, but with a different concept.

Premature contact, one of the occlusal diseases, occurs when one or two teeth come into contact first during occlusion. In addition, occlusion interference is when the teeth continue to touch during lateral movement. With these symptoms, people are apt to unconsciously grind or bit their teeth while sleeping.

Presently, to prevent this bad habit, a CBK Splint should be worn at bedtime. The standard centric relation splint was temporarily used by patients with poor temporomandibular joints, but the CBK Splint was designed and manufactured so that simultaneous occlusion would occur in the centric position where the skull is comfortable (maxilla and mandible are the most comfortable).

First, for ideal occlusion, use an occlusal analysis device called 'T-scan' to create the most ideal occlusion shape, and to compensate for the additional shortcomings. Skull balance occlusion stabilization helps to match the maximal intercuspal position in centric relation. When wearing this device, the masticatory muscles receive the minimum force (12 kg/cm^2).

If there is premature contact or lateral bite interference during occlusion, distortion occurs in the masticatory muscles, causing them to see a strong force of about 6~10 times greater than normal. Because of this, occlusal diseases such as cervical abrasion, attrition, hypersensitive teeth, tooth shaking, cracked teeth, destruction of alveolar bone, muscle pain, arthralgia, and joint noise may occur during sleep.

To prevent this, the CBK Splint using a 1.5 mm-thick metal strip bite was created as a skull-balanced occlusal splint. The device should be worn while sleeping or exercising to minimize occlusal force. When the occlusal force is lessened, the 22-bone skull and temporomandibular joints are stabilized. The wearing of this device greatly improves periodontal disease, and the quality of sleep is also improved.

There are many cases in which incurable diseases such as facial asymmetry, rhinitis, tinnitus, and migraine are also improved in clinical practice. This is because the device has the effect of increasing the amount of blood flowing to the brain. Furthermore, by further analyzing these phenomena, we are researching ways to prevent dementia that can occur due to lack of blood in the brain.

When a CBK Splint is combined with the 5 components of whole-body health including correct spine posture, abdominal breathing, mind control, eating and exercise, overall health can be improved.

03 Expected outcomes with dental treatment using CBK Splints

The CBK Splint is an intraoral device customized to fit the dental structure of each individual. It is a kind of stabilizing device modeled after the meshing of teeth with a metal strip bite[1)] in the posterior region where occlusion is adjusted.

The centric relation is the most important concept in not only dental health but also in whole-body health. The centric relation is a state in which the relationship between the upper and lower jaws is comfortable regardless of the teeth. That is, when the masseter muscle, temporal muscle, and medial pterygoid muscle contract in a stable temporomandibular joint state, the inferior belly of the lateral pterygoid muscle is completely relaxed. When the maximal intercuspal position (M.I) occurs at the same time in the centric relation (C.R), the occlusal force acts on the teeth, skull, and spine with minimal force.

To create this condition, the occlusal time is adjusted to within 0.3 seconds and the disclusion time to within 0.4 seconds using a T-scan. Then, to compensate for the lack of a little bit harmony, a CBK Splint should be worn while sleeping or exercising. When wearing a CBK Splint, centric relation (C.R) =

1) Metal strip bite that has been invented and patented with a thickness of 1.5 mm

the maximal intercuspal position (M.I), which is adjusted to a state where the occlusal force acts as a minimum of 12 ㎏/㎠, and the temporomandibular joint is also in an ideal state where the force is low.

▼ Comparison of Physiological functions and Non-physiological functions

Elements	Physiological function (orthofunction)	Non-physiological function parafunction (bruxism clenching)
Occlusal force	12 ㎏/㎠	74 ㎏/㎠
Contact mandibular position of teeth	Intercuspal position	Intercuspal position, eccentric position
Tooth contact time	15~20 minutes/day	2~162 minutes/day
condition of the muscles	Physiological	Unphysiological
Presence or absence of protective reflex	Presence	Absence
Impact of Affective Change	No impact	Impact

The differences between CBK Splints and conventional splints are as follows.

(1) CBK Splints have specialized 1.5 ㎜-thick metal strip bite.

(2) CBK Splints incorporate new concepts for intraoral treatment

such as occlusal adjustment.

(3) Benefits of occlusion has been extended to whole-body health with CBK Splints and spinal exercises.

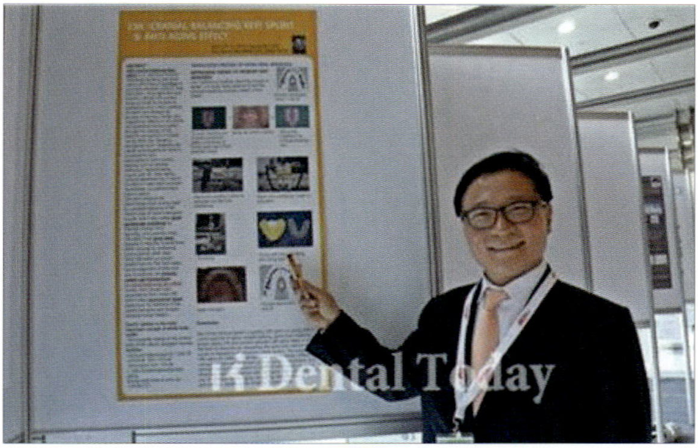

▲ Fig 7. Director Choi Byungkee standing in front of his poster

When subjected to destructive occlusal forces, distortion of the spine and skull occurs. And because of these distortions, aging occurs. CBK Splint can be one way to address the aging process.

The effects of the CBK Splint are endless. Although it is a simple device, the concept and method inherent in the actual CBK Splint are not simple. The effects this device has on the body are astonishing. A summary of them is as follows.

(1) The CBK Splint prevents teeth from further deterioration by addressing the destructive force of dental occlusal action.

While periodontal disease can be caused by improper brushing, the situation is made even worse by misalignment of the occlusion. Occlusal interference causes many diseases such as periodontal disease, cervical abrasion, and cracked teeth. It is subconsciously remembered and manifests itself as tooth clenching or bruxism during the night. Presently, the unphysiological masticatory force acting on the masticatory muscles is 74 kg/cm^2, which is more than six times the physiological occlusal force. As a result, there is tooth abrasion and the cervical region becomes worn, and teeth can crack. Also, complex problems such as abnormality in the temporomandibular joint and accelerated periodontal disease can occur. In particular, during sleep, grinding of teeth or swallowing movements (swallowing saliva or food) are performed once a minute. In the case of adults with severe tooth abrasion, an occlusal force of 6 to 10 times or more is applied, causing destruction to teeth and the periodontium. In this case, wearing a CBK Splint relieves the occlusal force and can prevent any further adverse effects on the teeth.

(2) People can sleep much deeper when they wear a CBK Splint. During sleep, a person performs a swallowing exercise to stimulate the brain by swallowing saliva. Adults with severe tooth wear cannot sleep deeply because their teeth and surrounding tissues are constantly stimulated by too much force when they swallow

saliva. This is one of the reasons why you can't sleep deeply as you get older. The CBK Splint relieves the force when swallowing, leading to a much more comfortable sleep.

(3) When a CBK Splint is worn, traction force is applied to the first (atlas) and second (axis) cervical vertebrae to help correct the arrangement of the spine. As a result, abnormal symptoms of the cranial nerve and cerebrospinal fluid caused by a fine twist of the 1st and 2nd cervical vertebrae are restored. The central axis of mandibular rotation when opening and closing the mouth is between the first and second cervical vertebrae. Occlusal interference occurs as the teeth wear down, and as the occlusal height decreases, and the cervical vertebrae become distorted. In addition, the temporomandibular joint directly and indirectly affects 68 muscles on the left and right sides.

According to C.M.Guzay, malocclusion of the teeth directly affects the temporomandibular joint and spine. If your spine in the right posture and you wear an occlusal splint, your spine will be straight, and your autonomic nerves will function normally. When the spine is straight, immunity is boosted. When the spine is upright, all immune cells (T cells, B cells, NK cells) can respond immediately. Conversely, if the spine is distorted, blood pressure rises and many incurable diseases such as tinnitus and rhinitis can develop. The cause of curvature of the spine is twisting of the cervical vertebrae due to bad posture and dental occlusion abnormalities. Therefore, correct posture and dental occlusion stabilization are essential conditions for spinal health.

(4) Facial asymmetry is alleviated, and the shape of the face becomes beautiful, and the balance of hormones is found by stabilizing the pituitary gland. If there is occlusion interference in the posterior teeth, 7~8 times the normal muscle distortion occurs in the masticatory muscles, the medial pterygoid and lateral pterygoid.

This distortion twists the sphenoid bone, which constitutes the very center of the skull composed of 22 bones. Most of the cranial nerves exit the sphenoid bone, and the pituitary gland above the sphenoid bone makes the body's hormones. As we age, our teeth become slightly distorted and wear away. This affects the sphenoid bone, resulting in facial asymmetry.

Therefore, wearing a CBK Splint restores facial asymmetry to some extent and helps smooth movement of hormones and cerebrospinal fluid.

The skull consists of 22 bones, which are bound together by sutures. As a person breathes, these sutures move through repeated flexion and extension. At that time, when the tooth cervical portion is subjected to a force sufficient to wear it down, the skull also receives the same force, causing sutureal jamming. This force deforms the temporal bone inward and outward, and also deforms the sphenoid bone, causing changes in the nervous system. It also contracts the muscles around the first (atlas) and second (axis) cervical vertebrae. This causes "atlas & axis subluxation," and the axis of the human body and the temporomandibular joint become distorted. Due to this small distortion, the entire spine is distorted in a domino effect. This in turn causes dural torque, and the cranial rhythmic impulse (C.R.I) is damaged, affecting the flow of cerebrospinal fluid. Furthermore, the nervous system and hormones are affected, resulting in various central and peripheral nerve diseases and hormonal diseases.

Occlusal adjustment using T-scan and the wearing of a CBK Splint can resolve these complex problems. The CBK Splint helps balance the autonomic nervous system and smooths the flow of hormones by stabilizing the skull and correcting the temporomandibular joint and spine. This has been said to be a key to protecting the whole-body health.

04 CBK Splint technology and manufacturing process

1 Occlusal adjustment with T-scan

Check the occlusal force of the patient's teeth on the left and right sides using a T-scan. By performing adjusting the occlusional adjustments, the occlusal force of the teeth is stabilized and by creating the most ideal tooth shapes are created.

2 Intraoral device manufacturing process

(1) Impressions : Impressions are made of the upper and lower jaws.

- Alginate (dental impression material) is used to make the impressions.

(2) Acquisition of Bites

- Patients are trained and practice swallowing exercises 3~4 times in which they swallow their saliva while placing their tongue on the roof of their mouth. Afterwards, my patented 1.5 ㎜ metal-coated occlusal check wax should be applied.

General Wax Bite

A general Wax Bite can identify the position of the intercuspation. However, it is difficult to have enough space to manufacture the splint. And it is difficult to take an accurate bite because of changes of the patient's biting force. Additionally, when manufacturing splints, there are many differences between the position on the articulator and the vertical dimension within the oral cavity.

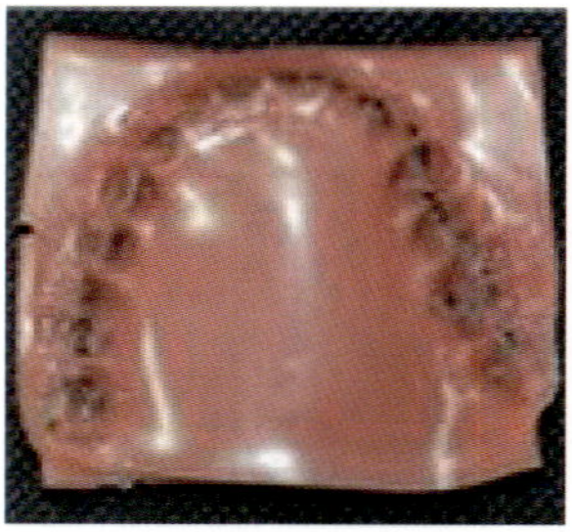

▲ Fig 8. General Wax Bite

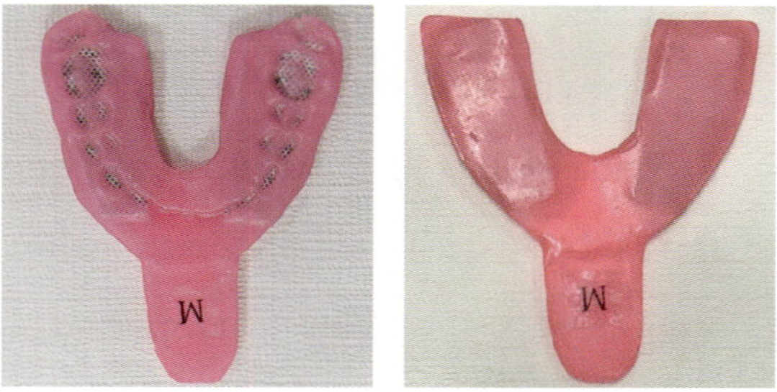

▲ Fig 9. Metal strip bite patented by Byungkee Choi

Wax Bite with metal strip

When the centric relation has been determined, the space necessary to manufacture a splint is readily available. It is easy to obtain an accurate bite, and differences in vertical dimension within the oral cavity can be reproduced on the articulator.

3 Development process of a 1.5 mm aluminum metal bite

1) At first, paraffin wax bite was used, but it failed.

Paraffin wax is the most commonly used material for getting bite registration in dentistry, and it allows the upper and lower jaw to naturally fit together to confirm centric occlusion. However, paraffin wax undergoes a lot of deformation during the process of mounting the model on the articulator, and errors are caused even when the desired thickness of 1.5 to 2 ㎜ is arbitrarily raised on the articulator.

In addition, there are cases where the occlusal stabilization appliance is greater than 2 ㎜. In the typical oral environment, when the upper and lower jaws are in a comfortable state, there is a gap called freeway space (a separation of 2~4 ㎜ when viewed from the anterior teeth). The CBK splint is designed in freeway space so that the patient will feel comfortable. If a thicker device than this is used, the muscles will be subjected to too much tensile force, which may be okay temporarily. But in the long run, it can cause harmful effects by inducing excessive tension in the temporomandibular joint. Likewise, if the thickness is less than 1.5 ㎜, the tensile force that stretches the temporomandibular joint will be less causing the device to be less effective and more likely to fracture.

Therefore, it is important to manufacture a device with a 1.5~2 ㎜ thick device, but the use of paraffin wax was discontinued due to the error caused by the wax bite, which requires the bite to be arbitrarily rasied on the articulator.

Many deformation errors are formed during the bite confirmation process after softening paraffin wax, due to the material itself softening and bending back and forth, left and right. And there were many inconsistencies between the actual model and the bite. For example, when combining a bite and impression model, force is applied across the wax bite to fix the model. In that situation, the wax itself is soft, so even if it is combined in the wrong direction, it is impossible to know this during the laboratory process. Under these conditions, many errors occur when the device is installed on a patient in an actual dental office. Therefore, even if the exact centric relation is recognized, it is not possible to secure the appropriate thickness (1.5~1.6 ㎜) desired in clinical practice during the splint manufacturing process. In addition, if the bite is arbitrarily raised to secure the articulator, the thickness of the occlusal surface of the posterior teeth can vary greatly from 2 ~7 ㎜, and the vertical and horizontal errors are large. Therefore, paraffin wax bite is no longer used.

2) Next, we used a trial and error method with a 1.5 mm (perforated hole) aluminum metal bite.

We evaluated perforated plate thicknesses of 0.4~5 mm, and perforated hole sizes of 0.7 mm and 1.5 mm. Initially, I used aluminum metal with 1.5 mm perforated holes and repeated trial and error by overlapping 1 to 3 pieces. When a 1.5 mm (perforated hole) aluminum metal bite was placed in the center and the wax was raised and lowered to create a bite, the deformation was significantly reduced compared to the existing wax bite and aluwax bite. Unfortunately, this also did not achieve the desired thickness of 1.5~2 mm, so this method was discontinued.

I placed two 1.5 mm (perforated hole) aluminum metal bites in the middle and apply wax up and down to register the bites. There is less distortion than when using just once piece. But it was difficult to obtain the desired thickness of 1.5~2 mm, so this method was also discontinued.

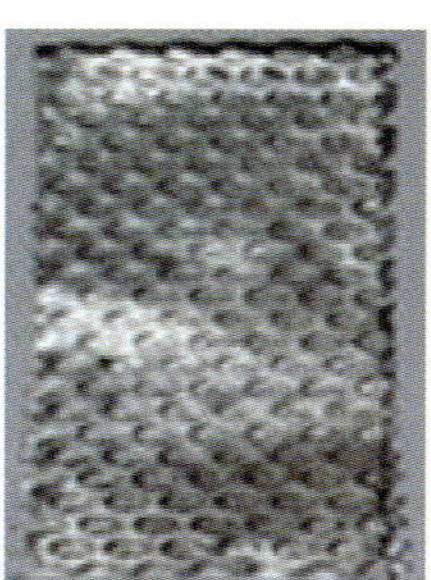

▲ Fig 10. 1.5 mm perforated hole aluminum

I placed three 1.5 mm (perforated hole) aluminum metal bites in the center and the wax was raised and lowered to register the bite. When I used metal bites with large perforated holes, there was a lot of distortion in patients with a large occlusal foce, so I stopped using them.

3) Finally success with a 0.7 mm (perforated hole) aluminum metal bite.

When I use two sheets of 0.7 ㎜ (perforated hole) aluminum metal bite coated with wax, there was deformation in cases where the patients had a large occlusal force. Since it was only about 1 ㎜ thick, it was difficult to achieve the appropriate splint thickness (1.5~2 ㎜), so it was discontinued. When I applied wax to three sheets of 0.7 ㎜ (perforated hole) aluminum metal bite, there was almost no deformation due to the occlusal pressure even in patients with strong occlusal force. And the bite was accurately recorded, ensuring the appropriate splint thickness (1.5~2.0 ㎜). This process was ultimately used based on the thickness of the bite.

I tried using a 1.5 ㎜ aluminum plate bite, but the wax was pushed out, so the bite did not registered well. In addition, bite deformation occurred as the wax surrounding the outer surface failed to bond and separated, so aluminum plates should not be used.

The appropriate splint thickness is about 1.5 to 2 ㎜ in the posterior region. The reason is that when the patient is in a comfortable state, there is about 1.5 to 2 ㎜ of freeway space in the posterior teeth. If it exceeds 4~5 ㎜ in posterior teeth, too much tensile force is applied to the temporomandibular joint, causing great discomfort and possibly causing temporomandibular joint disorders. If the thickness is less than 1.5~2.0 ㎜, the device may fracture and the splint will be less effective. Therefore, a splint with a thickness of 1.5 to 2 ㎜ is desirable. In addition, when registering a bite, if you overlap three pieces of 0.7 ㎜ perforated aluminum metal and apply wax to create a bite, so the upper and lower jaw will naturally be in the most comfortable position and a bite will be registered with the ideal centric relation. It plays a important role in the production of the centric relation appliance.

4) Structure of a 0.7 mm (perforated hole) aluminum metal bite

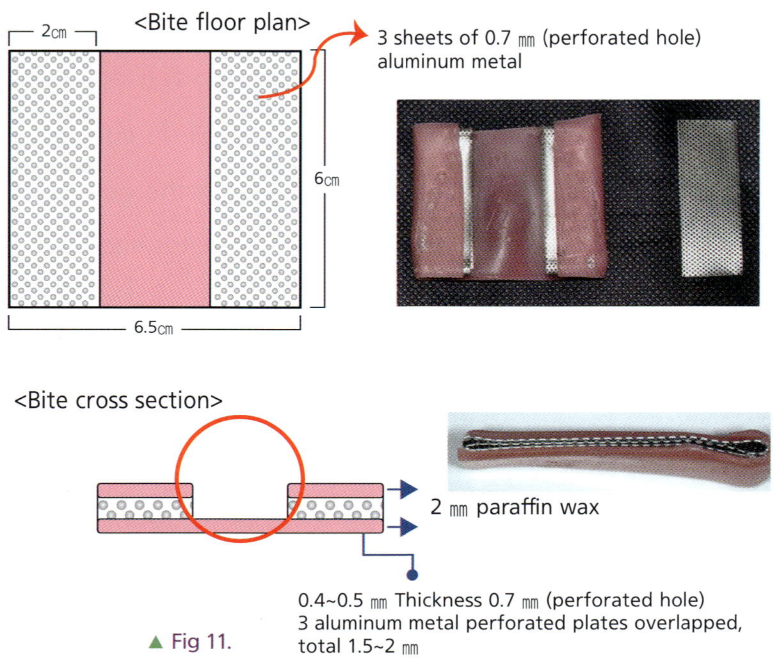

▲ Fig 11.

4 Treatment process and appliance manufacturing process

1) Registration of Bites

Patients are instructed to practice swallowing exercises 3 to 4 times by placing their tongue on the roof of their mouth and swallowing saliva. After that, wax should be applied to the 1.5 ㎜ metal-coated bite.

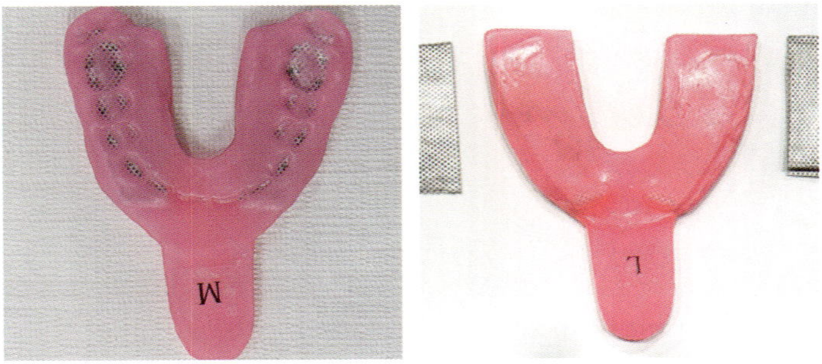

▲ Fig 12. Metal Strip Bite

2) Process of registering intraoral bites

The metal strip bite is made of 3 sheets of 0.7 ㎜ perforated aluminum metal strip (Thickness 0.4~0.5 ㎜). The total thickness is 1.5~2 ㎜. The role of the metal strip is to provide the necessary space of 1.5~2 ㎜ when manufacturing the splint and to act as a stopper to ensure the correct temporomandibular joint relationship.

3) Centric relation (CR) registration training procedure

① Frontmost position of the lower jaw: Bring the lower jaw forward as much as possible.

② Rearmost position of the lower jaw: Tuck the lower jaw back as much as possible.

③ Bite: Close slowly and stop when the first tooth touches.

④ Bite registration: Bite is taken in this state.

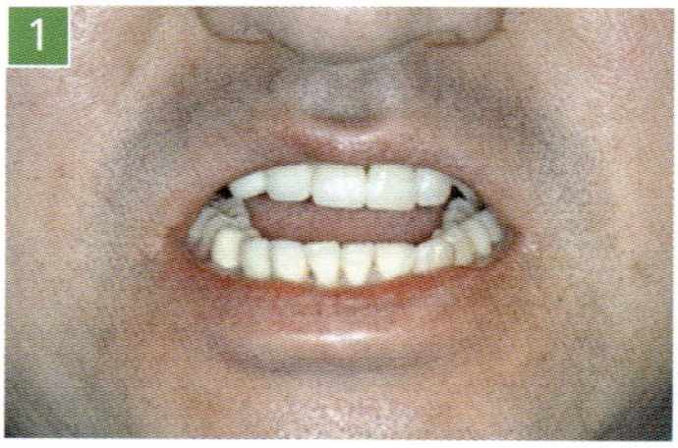

Mandibular most anterior position

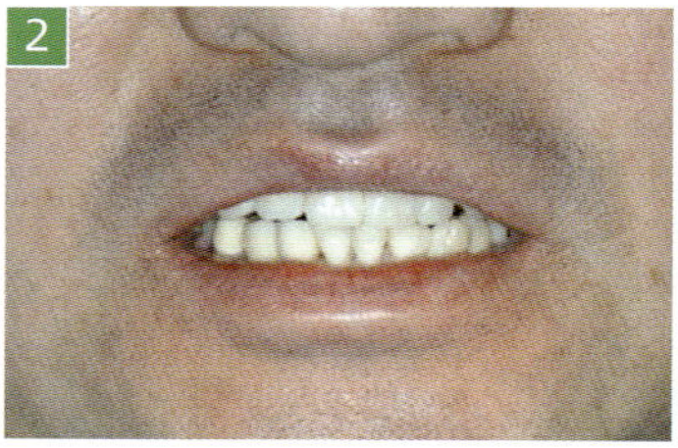

Mandibular most posterior position

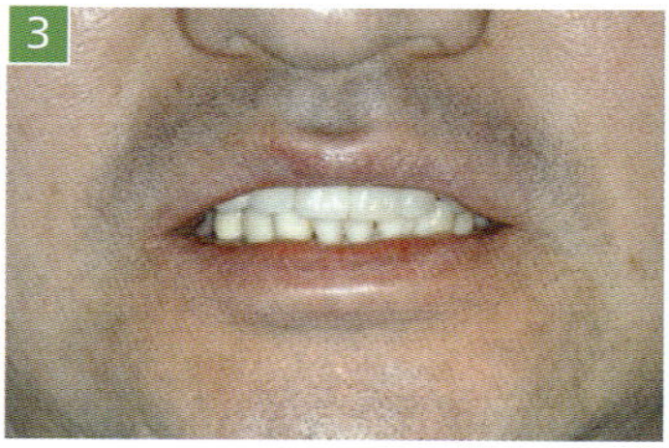

Bite

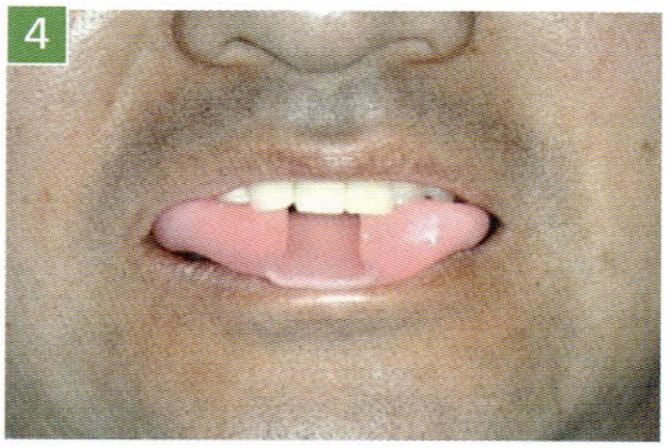

Bite registration

▲ Fig 13. Centric Relation(CR) registration training procedure

4) Registering a 0.7 mm (perforated hole) aluminum metal bite in the oral cavity

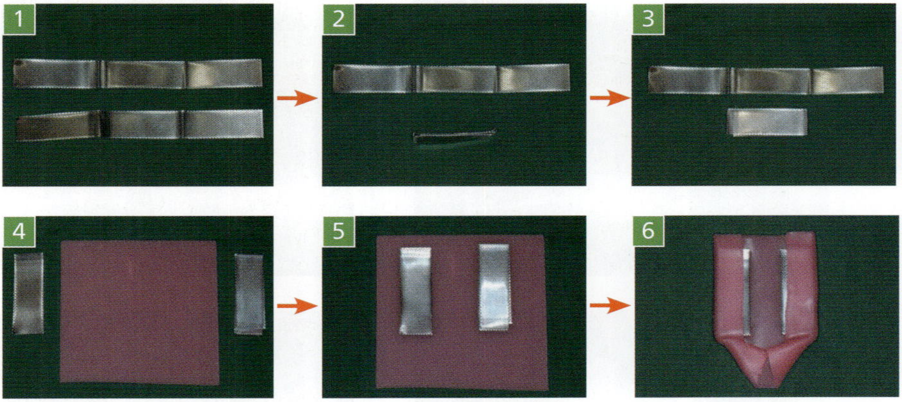
▲ Fig 14. 0.7 ㎜ (perforated hole) aluminum metal bite formation for intraoral registration

5) Mounting the maxillary model using the average value (sagittal condylar inclination, Bennett angle) on the articulator

A precise appliance is produced by mounting it on an articulator using the average value of the temporomandibular joint angle in the oral cavity.

6) Using a metal strip bite, mounting the mandibular model on the articulator

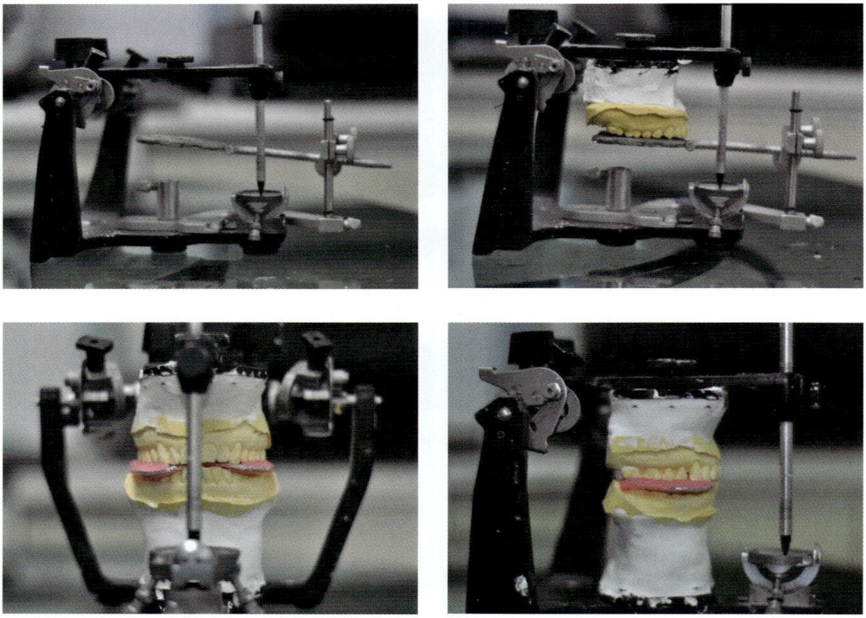

▲ Fig 15. Mounting the upper and lower jaw casts on the articulator

7) Surveyor work on the tooth model of the patient who is to wear the splint

Using a surveyor for dental technicians, determine the appropriate insertion path of the patient who is to wear the splint. Once the appropriate insertion path has been determined, fill undercut area on the insertion path with wax to ensure that the completed appliance can be inserted and removed smoothly.

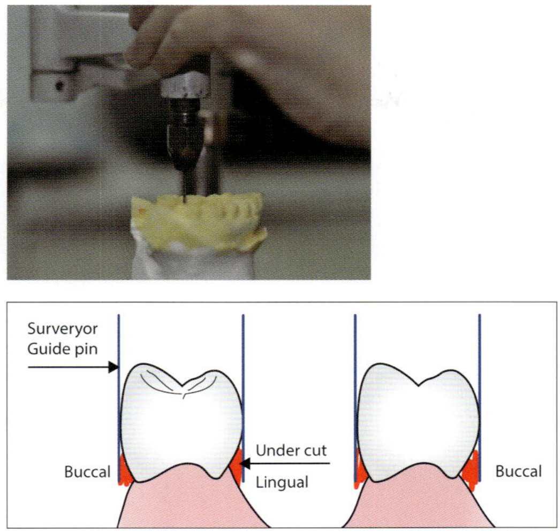

▲ Fig 16. Surveyor work on the tooth model of the patient who is to wear the splint

- What to watch: Observe the depressed area of the tooth, that is, the undercut area between the tooth and gums, using a surveyor guide pin.
- Observation results: It affects the insertion and removal of the splint into the oral cavity and the control of the retention force of the appliance.

8) Resin pouring and polymerization using polymerization machine

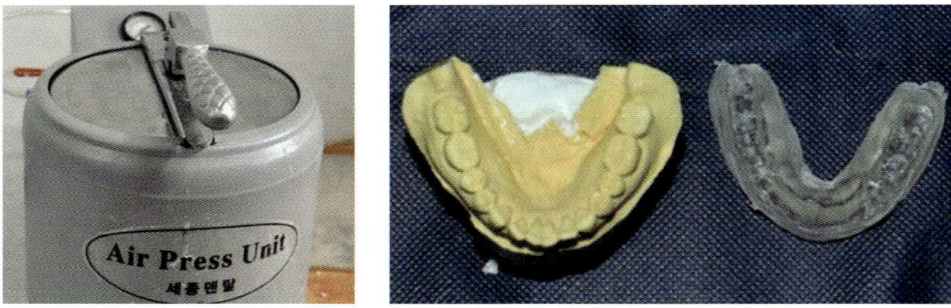

▲ Fig 17. Polymerization using resin pouring and polymerization machine

9) Trim splints and check occlusion

When checking occlusion, check that all teeth touch at one point and check canine guidance during lateral movement.

When checking occlusion, select a piece of articulating paper that allows you to check both sides at once. Select and confirm using 80 ㎛ and 40 ㎛ thick articulating papers.

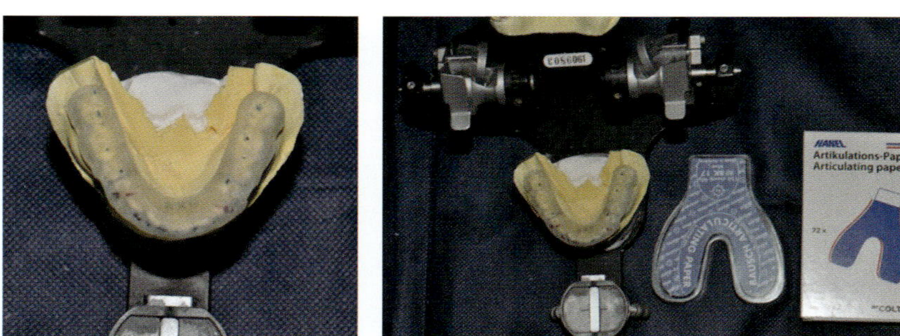

▲ Fig 18. Trim splints and check occlusion

When checking unilateral occlusion, the patient cannot bite into the exact CR position, so if possible, check both sides at once.

10) Finish the splint using dental abrasives

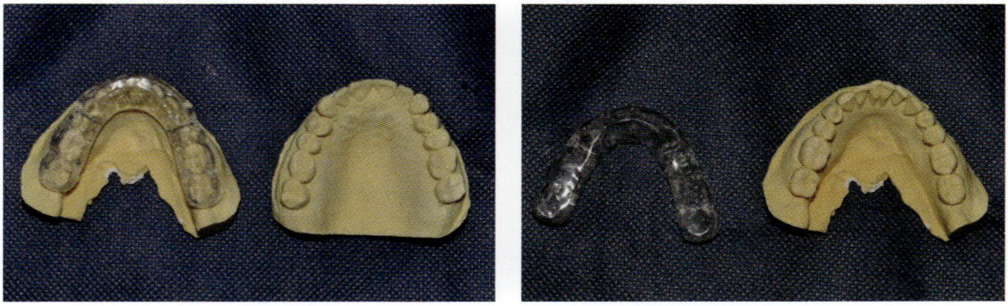

▲ Fig 19. Finish the splint using dental abrasives

Two or three adjustments will be needed over time, and changes in occlusion are inspected and corrected every three months. And after adjustment, polishing is done.

5 Comparison of omnivac splints and resin build-up splints

	Omnivac splint	Resin build-up splint
Advantages	• Easy to manufacture • Low cost	• Able to accurately replicate impressions • Retention can be adjusted • Possible correction in case of tooth deformation
Disdvantages	• Appliance retention capacity is low • There might be an error in the occlusal point because of the gap between the appliance and the teeth • Deformed teeth cannot be corrected • If resin is added when correcting occlusion, the resin often falls off or breaks over time • Difficult to repair, poor appliance retention	• Long production time • High production costs • The production process is complicated

6 Things to keep in mind during the manufacturing process

The CBK Splint is similar in shape to other splints, but the CBK Splint is manufactured by adjusting the bite to a thickness of

1.5~2 ㎜. The bite is made by overlapping three 0.4~0.5 ㎜ thick aluminum metal strips with a hole size of about 0.7 ㎜. Paraffin wax is applied on top to create a bite with a thickness of 1.5 to 2 ㎜.

Equipment called T-scan is used to accurately and reliably adjust occlusion before manufacturing the appliance. By adjusting the occlusion, the natural teeth must first be brought into an ideal shape, the occlusal force must be stabilized, and then the bite for the CBK Splint must be registered. When registering a bite, the patient's spine must be straight.

I manufacture CBK Splint with the bite I have acquired this way. Therefore, it is designed to help with systemic diseases of unknown cause such as migraine, tinnitus, rhinitis, high blood pressure, and disc herniation. These systematic diseases can be caused by asymmetry of the left and right temporomandibular joints that can occur due to changes in occlusion and subluxation of the first and second cervical vertebrae. When the lateral and medial pterygoid muscles become distorted due to changes in occlusion (due to wear and occlusal interference), the sphenoid bone at the center that the skull made up of 22 bones is deformed, causing problems with facial asymmetry and hormone secretion. However, this distortion of the sphenoid bone has been restored with a CBK Splint, which restored facial asymmetry and balanced hormonal secretion, thereby improving health.

Therefore, although the shape is similar to that of other

splints, the thickness of this device is different and the concept of treatment within the oral cavity, such as adjusting the occlusion of teeth, is completely different. Another feature is that it is linked to overall health through full-body exercises to straighten the spine after the appliance has been installed. A common belief is that the most important change in overall health (aging) is the distortion of the spine and skull due to a decrease in vertical dimension, thus the CBK Splint was invented as a solution.

When installing a splint in a patient's mouth, the temporomandibular joint must form an ideal relationship in centric relation. In addition, the teeth must form an ideal occlusion. Ideal occlusion occurs when the posterior teeth are each in equal contact with their opposing teeth, and the anterior teeth create a canine guidance (Dot in back line in front).

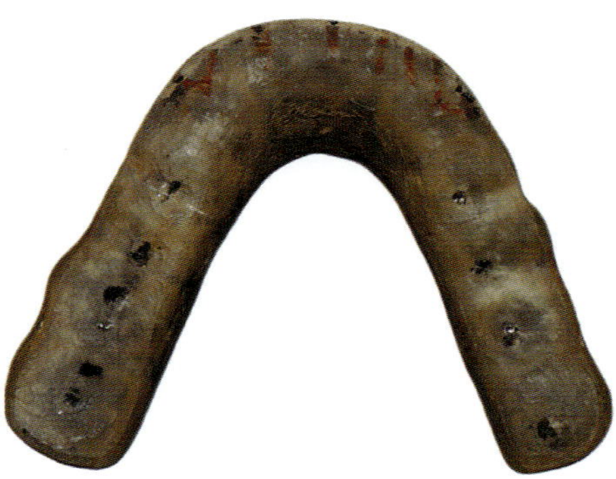

▲ Fig 20. CBK Splint occlusal adjustment

05 CBK Splints and FDA registration and government patents

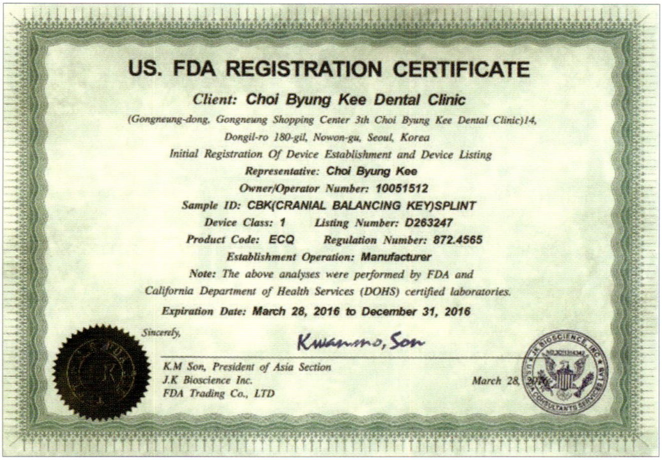

US. FDA REGISTRATION CERTIFICATE

Client: **Choi Byung Kee Dental Clinic**

(Gongneung-dong, Gongneung Shopping Center 3th Choi Byung Kee Dental Clinic)14, Dongil-ro 180-gil, Nowon-gu, Seoul, Korea

Initial Registration Of Device Establishment and Device Listing

Representative: **Choi Byung Kee**

Owner/Operator Number: **10051512**

Sample ID: **CBK(CRANIAL BALANCING KEY)SPLINT**

Device Class: **1** *Listing Number:* **D263247**

Product Code: **ECQ** *Regulation Number:* **872.4565**

Establishment Operation: **Manufacturer**

Note: The above analyses were performed by FDA and California Department of Health Services (DOHS) certified laboratories.

Expiration Date: **March 28, 2016 to December 31, 2016**

Sincerely,

Kwanmo, Son

K.M Son, President of Asia Section
J.K Bioscience Inc.
FDA Trading Co., LTD

March 28, 20

▲ Fig 21. CBK Splint, US FDA Registration Certificate

1 CBK Splint registered with US FDA

The CBK (Cranial Balancing Key) Splint, a cranial balancing occlusal stabilizer, recognized globally. The CBK Splint received a registration certificate from the U.S. FDA and the California Department of Health Services (DOHS) as a Medical Devices Class 1 grade, listing number D263247, and product code ECQ on March 26, 2016.

The CBK splint is a appliance that is placed in the mouth while the wearer sleeps or exercises. It is a medical device that improves overall health by maintaining not only dental health but also the balance of the cerebrum, spine, nervous system, and hormones that are connected to dental occlusion.

Other splints have been mainly used to protect the temporomandibular joint and teeth, but the CBK splint goes one step further and is a centric relation occlusal stabilization splint to improve overall health.

The CBK splint is a 'stabilizer that plays a important role in maintaining the balance of the skull.' It creates a comfortable relationship between the upper and lower jaw by first adjusting the occlusion of the teeth and then perfectly adjusting the missing parts.

2 CBK Splint domestic patent registration

The 'CBK Splint' received an invention patent from the Korean Intellectual Property Office on May 6, 2015.

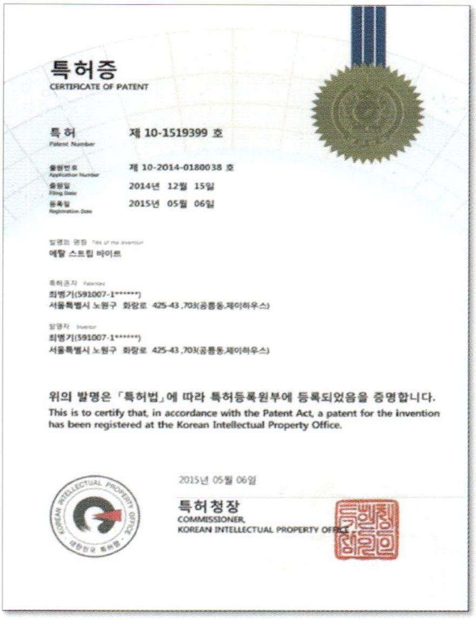

특허증
CERTIFICATE OF PATENT

특허 Patent Number 제 10-1519399 호

출원번호 Application Number 제 10-2014-0180038 호
출원일 Filing Date 2014년 12월 15일
등록일 Registration Date 2015년 05월 06일

발명의 명칭 Title of the Invention
메탈 스트립 바이트

특허권자 Patentee
최병기(591007-1******)
서울특별시 노원구 화랑로 425-43 ,703(공릉동,제이하우스)

발명자 Inventor
최병기(591007-1******)
서울특별시 노원구 화랑로 425-43 ,703(공릉동,제이하우스)

위의 발명은 「특허법」에 따라 특허등록원부에 등록되었음을 증명합니다.
This is to certify that, in accordance with the Patent Act, a patent for the invention has been registered at the Korean Intellectual Property Office.

2015년 05월 06일

특허청장
COMMISSIONER,
KOREAN INTELLECTUAL PROPERTY OFFICE

▲ Fig 22. CBK Splint patent certificate

The CBK Splint has received international recognition by being registered with the U.S. FDA and obtaining a patent in Korea. We plan to spread this beneficial technology to many countries around the world, including the United States and China.

06 Future developments for the CBK Splint

Since we developed the CBK Splint and started installing it on patients, we have had more than 5,000 clinical cases at our dental hospital alone.

The author educates patients visiting the hospital by emphasizing that wearing CBK splints, correcting spine posture, abdominal breathing, proper diet and exercise, and a positive mindset are important for human immunity. The author became convinced of these concepts after seeing patients whose overall health recovered after using CBK Splints, so he organized the theories and presented them to the International College of Prosthodontists(ICP) under the title "Anti-aging effect of CBK Splints." In addition, we lecture at specialized dental seminars for dentists, which are attracting attention from dentists.

In the future, we plan to expand the use of CBK Splints and collect additional clinical evidence of their various effects through joint research with doctors from many other departments, including internal medicine, otolaryngology, neurology, orthopedics, and oriental medicine. In addition, based on the fact that the splints can have a positive effect on preventing dementia by increasing blood flow to the brain, we plan to verify the results based on evidence from more than 5,000 cases treated directly at our hospital.

In addition, by applying some of the latest manufacturing technologies such as 3D printers, we aim to innovate ways to make our splints more precise and suitable for each individual's tooth structure. If mass production becomes possible through innovation in manufacturing technology, it is expected that the unit cost of splint manufacturing will be reduced, thereby lowering the burden on patients.

The CBK Splint received a patent from the Korean Intellectual Property Office in 2015 as a creative invention under the name 'Metal Strip Bite'. And in 2016, it was registered as a 'Medical Device' by the US FDA and DOHS (California Department of Health Services).

In addition, it received awards in five categories, including a gold award and a special award from the organizer, at the World Invention Competition held in Toronto, Canada on August 26, 2023. This is further evidence that the theoretical background and effectiveness of CBK Splint are recognized globally.

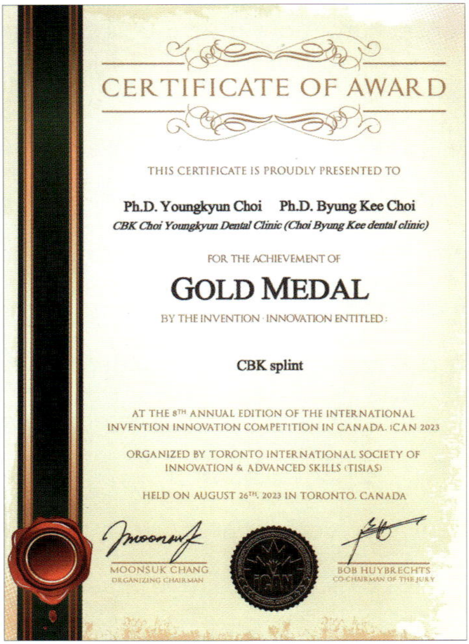
CERTIFICATE OF AWARD

THIS CERTIFICATE IS PROUDLY PRESENTED TO

Ph.D. Youngkyun Choi Ph.D. Byung Kee Choi

CBK Choi Youngkyun Dental Clinic (Choi Byung Kee dental clinic)

FOR THE ACHIEVEMENT OF

GOLD MEDAL

BY THE INVENTION · INNOVATION ENTITLED :

CBK splint

AT THE 8TH ANNUAL EDITION OF THE INTERNATIONAL INVENTION INNOVATION COMPETITION IN CANADA. iCAN 2023

ORGANIZED BY TORONTO INTERNATIONAL SOCIETY OF INNOVATION & ADVANCED SKILLS (TISIAS)

HELD ON AUGUST 26TH, 2023 IN TORONTO, CANADA

MOONSUK CHANG
ORGANIZING CHAIRMAN

BOB HUYBRECHTS
CO-CHAIRMAN OF THE JURY

▲ Fig 23. Gold medal certificate

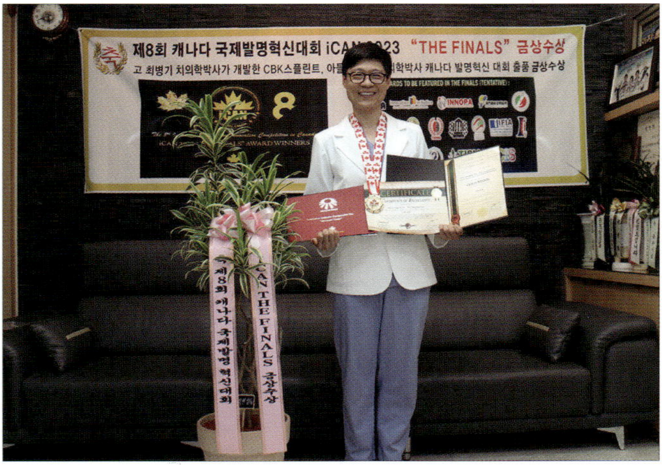
제8회 캐나다 국제발명혁신대회 iCA
023 "THE FINALS" 금상수상
고 최병기 치의학박사가 개발한 CBK스플린트, 아들
의학박사 캐나다 발명혁신 대회 출품 금상수상
제8회 캐나다 국제발명 혁신대회
iCAN THE FINALS 금상수상

▲ Fig 24. Dr. Choi Youngkyun received the certificate

Based on technological prowess recognized in the Republic of Korea and abroad, we plan to expand its distribution to the rest of the world, including the United States and Europe, starting with Japan, China, and Southeast Asia, which have many similarities with Korea.

Just as nobody can live today for even a moment without a smartphone, it is my humble dream to see people all over the world enjoying a healthy and happy life by wearing a CBK Splint every night.

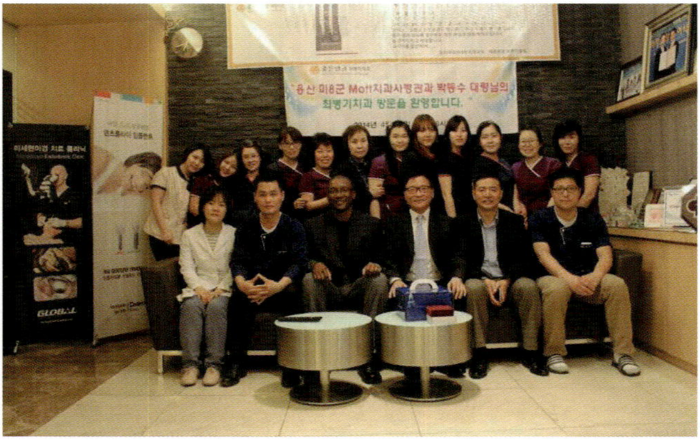

▲ Fig 25. Colonel Park Dong-soo, commander of Mott Dental, 8th U.S. Army, Yongsan, and dental staff at Dr. Byungkee Choi Dental Clinic

chapter 03

Dental Clinical Effects of CBK Splints

01 Helps to perfect occlusion

02 Reduces the need for tooth extraction

03 Protects the occlusion adjusted by T-Scan

04 Supports a harmonious masticatory system

05 Maintains a 'centric relation' as the keyword in dental treatment

06 Reduces occlusal diseases

07 Increases the implant success rate

08 Increases facial asymmetry treatment effects

09 Protects teeth and stabilizes dentition

01 Helps to perfect occlusion

1 Importance of occlusion

The main cause of tooth loss is trauma, but occlusal interference, premature contact on one side before the other side during occlusion (tooth meshing), is also a major cause. Another major cause is microorganisms such as bacteria, viruses, and fungi. Considering these three factors, if the occlusal force is controlled and germs are prevented, teeth can be maintained in their current state for life.

So this raises the question, between 'occlusion force' and 'bacteria,' which one causes more damage to teeth?

Back in 1917, Stillman stated that occlusion was more damaging to teeth than germs. After that and until the 1970s, it was thought that bacteria remaining on teeth due to poor brushing was the biggest cause of tooth loss. Then, in the 1980s, with the development of EMG (electronic muscle force measuring device) that measures muscle strength, the action of the masticatory muscles was better understood, and it was concluded that abnormal occlusion was 2~4 times more harmful to teeth than bacteria. Boston dentists Harrel and Nunn published a groundbreaking paper on this in 2009.

Currently, world-renowned dentist Peter Dawson has said, "Occlusal congestion is the biggest cause of tooth loss. Occlusal disease is far more devastating than tooth decay or periodontal disease," and "only 2 % of dentists understand and treat occlusion."

If there is premature contact while sleeping at night, the occlusal force increases. In addition, during lateral movement, if there is an area where the teeth come into contact first, a lot of occlusal force is applied. During sleep, swallowing movements are performed once a minute, and teeth clenching, or bruxism, occurs to compensate for this abnormal contact. Because of this, occlusal tooth disease is common.

Therefore, it is important to maintain proper occlusion starting at a young age by evaluating the occlusion at each visit to the dentist and performing fine occlusion adjustments while continuing oral care through scaling. When occlusion is not good, prosthetics, orthodontics, and oral surgery should be considered for ideal occlusion, and a CBK Splint should be considered as an alternative option.

■ Posterior occlusal interference

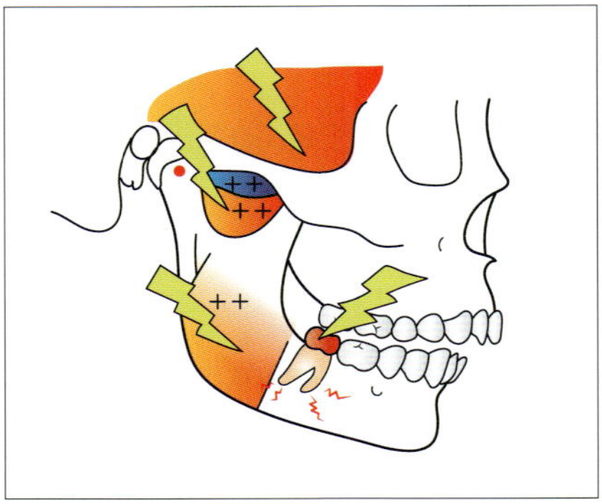

▲ Fig 26. Posterior occlusion interference[2)]

During mandibular movement, if there is occlusal interference in any molar, the lateral pterygoid muscle becomes activated and the arrector muscle is overactivated. This causes excessive muscle activity due to incongruity and gives a strong horizontal force to the posterior teeth, resulting in the risk of damaging them. This force easily causes excessive tooth articulation, fracture, and excessive tooth movement.

In order to resolve this problem of occlusion, implement the method presented by the author at the 16th International College of Prosthodontists. As the initial step, the occlusion should be adjusted to slightly correct the teeth to the occlusion form of youth using a T-scan.

2) Peter. E. Dawson(2012), *Functional Occlusion : From TMJ to Smile Design*, Philadelphia, PA, USA, MOSBY ELSEVIER, ISBN-9780323033718. p.67

In the second step, CBK Splints are used to resolve excessive occlusion force for those who have difficulty obtaining an ideal occlusion through occlusal adjustment. The CBK Splint is a type of centric relation night guard. In my hospital, more than 5,000 patients have used CBK Splints, and most of them have shown satisfactory results in terms of teeth, gums, and general health.

For the final step, currently, when bite force is too great, Botox is injected into the masticatory muscles (specifically into the masseter and temporalis muscles) once every 3~4 months to contract them. In this way, the masticatory force can be weakened to about 60 % of the original state.

In summary, the problems of high occlusal force are resolved by 1) occlusion adjustment, 2) wearing a CBK splint, and 3) Botox injection.

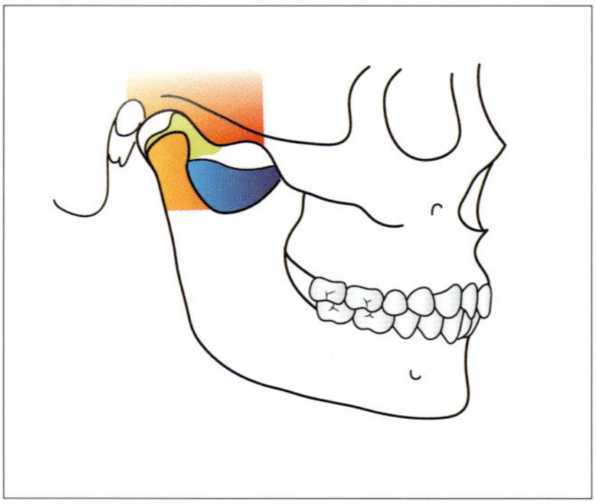

▲ Fig 27. A perfect occlusion that meets all criteria for success is remarkably stable, requiring only minimal adjustments over many years.

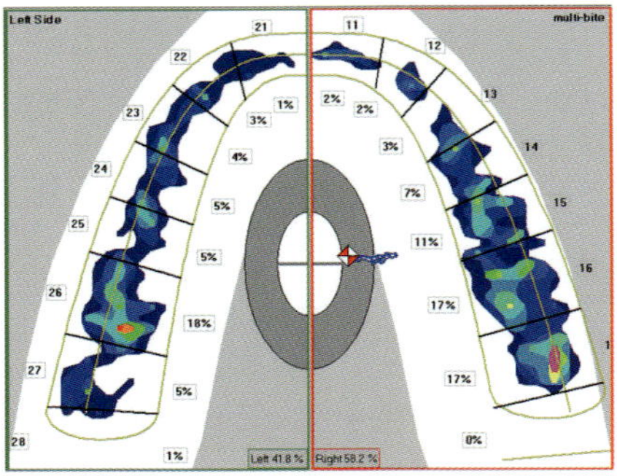

▲ Fig 28. An occlusal device made according to the ideal occlusal standard can maintain good dental and periodontal health.

In order to cope with bacterial problems, it is desirable to take care of the gingiva every 3 months for adults who brush their teeth well but have poor gingiva, while for the general population, scaling should be done once every 6 months. In addition, for patients with severe gingiva disease, bacteria are managed through probiotics lactic acid bacteria and a powder called Exoden.

2 Occlusal analysis & occlusal adjustment

1) Occlusal Analysis

Occlusal analysis is a study of the contact surfaces where the upper and lower teeth meet and the factors that affect the structures related to the occlusal surface. Let's find out what to look for when performing occlusal analysis.

① Centric contact point

How a centric stop occurs is analyzed in the centric relation (CR).

② Premature contact in centric relationship

An impression of the teeth is taken to make a master cast of the tooth shapes and positions so premature contacts can be located on the master cast. Presently, it is easy to find premature contacts using a T-scan.

③ Working side contact

When performing lateral movements to one side, the canines do the main work while the rest of the teeth are immediately discluded. With age, tooth wear occurs, so during lateral movement, the first and second premolars and first molars may come into contact. When this happens and there is excessive contact during lateral movement, muscle distortion may occur, which applies excessive force to the temporomandibular joint. Consequently, traumatic occlusion might occur.

④ Balancing side contact

If food is chewed on just one side, the lingual cusp (the raised part of the tooth where the upper and lower teeth engage each other) of the second molar on the opposite side may get caught. When this happens, subconsciously, efforts are made to compensate to resolve the occlusion interference of the second molars. In particular, for this compensatory task, when swallowing once a minute while sleeping, by clenching or grinding teeth, the surrounding muscles receive 6~10 times more force than usual. As a result, muscle distortion occurs, resulting in occlusal diseases such as cervical abrasion, hypersensitivity, attrition (wearing away teeth), and cracked teeth.

⑤ Protrusive contact

When the mandible moves anteriorly, there should be harmonious contact between the anterior teeth. If the anterior teeth come into contact with just one tooth, the temporomandibular joint and masticatory muscles become distorted; therefore, anterior limit movement and harmonious forward contact are important.

⑥ Aspects of wear (attrition)

Abrasion means there is premature contact or occlusal interference, so occlusal adjustment and splint treatment are necessary.

⑦ Changes in the vertical dimensions of occlusion

Changes in occlusal dimensions due to wear should be addressed. If there is premature contact or occlusal interference, muscles, sutures of the skull, and the teeth become distorted (sutural jamming). It should be recognized that these phenomena can also affect the nervous system and hormones.

⑧ Irregularities of the occlusal plane

There should be no traumatic occlusion due to premature

contact or occlusal interference when the plane of occlusion has a harmonious curve (Curve of Wilson, Curve of Spee) in front and back or left and right.

2) Three conditions for stable occlusion

Stable occlusion can be realized when the following three conditions are met:

① The temporomandibular joint must be comfortable and healthy. Premature tooth contact or occlusal interference can cause muscle pain due to muscle distortion, and in severe cases, displacement of the joint disc occurs. In more severe cases, there may be degenerative changes in the joints. Therefore, the most important thing is that the mandibular condyle should be in the centric relation and located in the foremost position in the glenoid fossa. Dental treatment should start with a healthy temporomandibular joint.

② When guiding the mandible anteriorly, it must remain within the limit motion. Without anterior guidance of the anterior teeth, the posterior teeth receive much more force.

③ The maximal intercuspation (MI) must occur in the centric relation (CR) state. To accomplish this, I use a T-scan, a measuring instrument, to measure the occlusal force hourly and perform occlusal adjustment. If it is still not perfect, I prescribe that a CBK Splint be worn at night to match the centric relation and the maximal intercuspal position for minimal occlusal force.

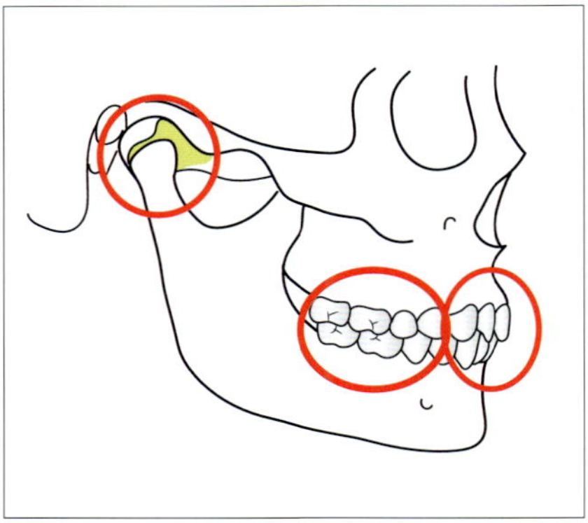

▲ Fig 29. successful occlusal treatment

3) Occlusion Equilibrium

Occlusal equilibrium refers to the elimination of biased occlusal contact that interferes with the physical function of the temporomandibular joint, that is, elimination of early contact or occlusal interference.

As viewed from the front, the left and right occlusion should be evenly aligned, and as viewed from the side, the occlusion should be even. When simultaneous occlusion (maximum cusp interlocking position) is matched in the centric relation, physiological occlusion occurs and the muscles act with the minimum force (12 ㎏/㎠).

A balancing interference is when the rearmost tooth on the opposite side becomes caught when chewing food is done on one side. Presently, occlusal diseases such as pain in the temporomandibular joint, abrasion of the dental cervical region, abrasion, hypersensitivity, and alveolar bone destruction may occur, and migraines, shoulders, and back may also be present. In this case, it can be seen clinically that the symptoms disappear with occlusal adjustment.

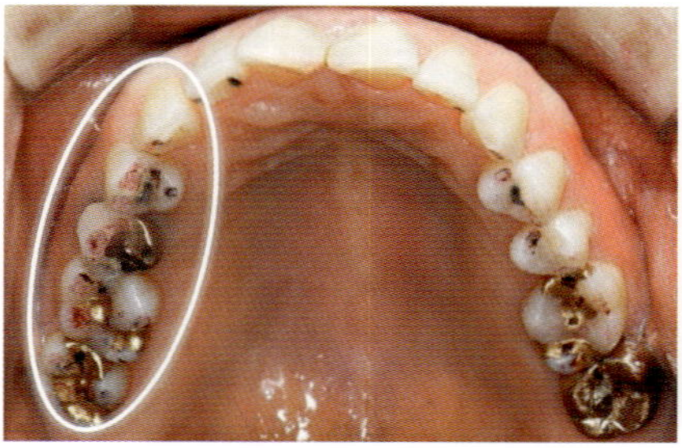

▲ Fig 30. Before occlusal adjustment

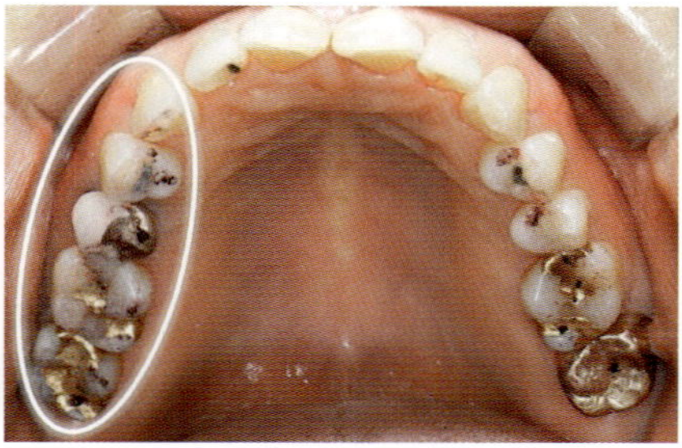

▲ Fig 31. After occlusal adjustment

Once there is no disorder upon opening or no degenerative change at the time of the temporomandibular joint examination, about 85 % of temporomandibular joint patients with muscle discomfort can be treated with occlusal adjustment.

However, if the articular disc is missing or the temporomandibular joint has degenerative changes, it is necessary to stabilize the temporomandibular joint through physical therapy or splint treatment before adjusting the occlusion. In the past, the occlusion was adjusted by taking an impression of the patient's oral cavity, making a master cast, and using it to plan the adjustments in advance. Unfortunately, this was difficult, but currently, the time and force of the occlusal contact point can be easily adjusted using an occlusal analysis device called T-scan.

4) Correction of Occlusal Incongruity

If there is any premature contact in which one tooth touches first, or occlusal interference, that is, when the teeth behind the canines receive more force than the canines when eating on one side, the teeth receive undue force, resulting in occlusal diseases such as cervical abrasion, attrition, temporomandibular joint disorder, and muscle pain.

If the mismatch of the occlusion is large, the teeth can be corrected, and the teeth can be realigned. In addition, prosthetic treatment or oral surgery can significantly reposition the dentition. If the temporomandibular joint is disease-free and there is just a small occlusal mismatch, occlusion adjustment can adjust the teeth into a younger form, but if there is occlusal disease, a CBK Splint should be worn during sleep to keep the centric relation and maximal intercuspal position, maintaining a comfortable state with minimal force on the teeth and skull.

Even if orthodontic treatment or two-jaw surgery is performed, there are many cases where the centric relation and maximal intercuspal position do not match. In this case, occlusion adjustment and CBK Splint treatment are used to keep the dentition from misaligning any further.

02 Reduces the need for tooth extraction

1 The largest reason for tooth extraction

According to Dawson, there are two major causes of tooth extraction, and this is also true for implant patients. The first is stress due to trauma or occlusion (meshing of teeth), while the second is periodontal disease caused by microorganisms such as bacteria, viruses, and fungi. Therefore, if both occlusal forces and bacteria can be controlled, the implant can be maintained for a lifetime.

In 1917, American dentist Stillman first announced that teeth need to be extracted due to poor occlusion rather than bacteria. After that, in the 1950s, 60s, and 70s, scholars conducted a lot of research on the importance of occlusion and bacteria in tooth preservation using animals such as monkeys and dogs and cadavers. During this period, it was announced that most of the teeth were extracted because of bacteria rather than poor occlusion.

However, since the 1990s, studies have focused on occlusal abnormalities being a greater cause of tooth damage and the need for tooth extractions than bacteria.

In 1992, Burgett showed the importance of occlusion by publishing a paper that showed recovery from gingiva disease was much faster in his treatment group in which occlusal adjustment was concurrent with bacteria control with gingiva treatment than in the group with only bacteria control with gingiva treatment. In addition, in 2009, Boston dentists Harrel and Nunn published an important and groundbreaking paper stating that in patients with abnormal dental occlusion (i.e., premature contact or excessive contact of teeth other than the canines during lateral movement of the mandible) periodontal pocket depth was 2~4 times worse than in those with just poor oral hygiene who did not brush.

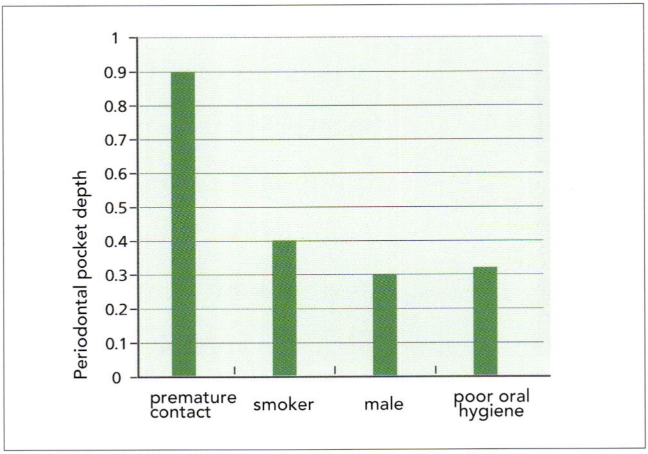

▲ Fig 32. Effects of periodontal pocket growth in early contact compared to smoking, gender, and poor oral hygiene status. –Harrel and Nunn, 2009 –

World-renowned prosthodontist Robert. B. Kerstein and Radke J. published a paper in 2012 that proposed that the greatest cause of TMD (Temporo-Mandibular Joint Disorder) is a function of the "working side." In addition, Mark A. Piper's paper in 2013 stated that the greater the 'slide in centric' in the centric relation, the greater the detrimental effect on the temporomandibular joint. From this, it can be seen that improper occlusion is the largest cause of TMD. According to paper, when the teeth are finely misaligned, the facial muscles receive 6~10 times more force, and there are 7 other signs and symptoms such as tooth wear and cracked teeth, hypersensitivity, tooth mobility, repeated sounds, cervical wear, periodontitis, and arthralgia.

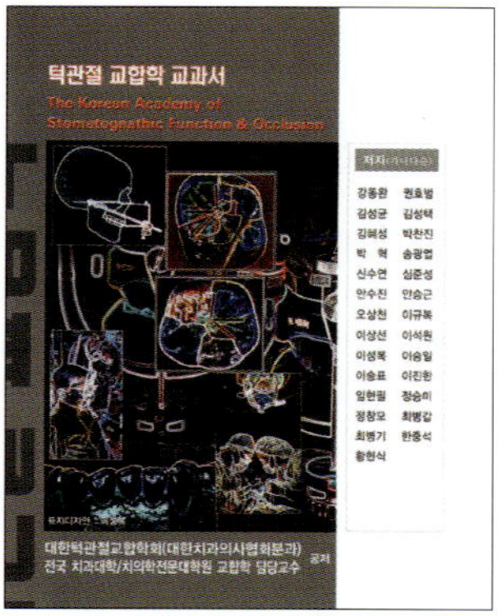

▲ Fig 33. Textbook of human jaw function & occlusion(2014)[3]

When a dentist discovers issues with the overall maxillofacial systems, it is important for the dentist to take preventive measures through diagnosis before the symptoms. I published this information in Textbook of human jaw function & occlusion in 2014.

3) Co-authored by professors in charge of occlusion at the Korean Temporomandibular Joint Occlusal Society's Graduate School of Dentistry (April 12, 2014), Temporomandibular joint occlusion textbook, Seoul: Yenang I&C

2 Solving the occlusion problem

To solve the problem of occlusion, it is necessary to start with occlusal adjustment. Occlusal abnormalities must first be restored to the form of youth by making a fine occlusion adjustment while the temporomandibular joint is maintained in a healthy state.

85 % of temporomandibular joint patients have muscle problems. In the case of 'muscle problems,' periodontal treatment is recommended and then an occlusal adjustment to remove premature contact in the centric relation and occlusal interference in the lateral position.

Although the T-scan III is most useful for diagnosing premature contact of occlusion and interference with occlusion, more than an 80 % accurate diagnosis can be made by an experienced dentist using only occlusion. However, if the position of the temporomandibular joint is distorted or degenerated, it is necessary to take a careful approach after stabilizing it with splint, muscle exercise, and drug therapy. People swallow saliva once a minute during sleep. At this time, if the teeth are high or crooked and do not fit well, the person will grind or clench their teeth to resolve this on their own.

If there is a lack of occlusal adjustment, the teeth must be preserved by wearing a CBK Splint, which is similar to an atheletic mouthpiece, while sleeping. The CBK Splint is similar in shape to a conventional splint, but the thickness of the device is different, and the concept of intraoral treatment, such as tooth occlusion adjustment, is different. Further more, its use is related to the health of the whole body through a whole-body exercise to straighten the spine after the device is installed. If a 1.5 ㎜ thick CBK Splint is worn during exercise other than sleeping, it induces stabilization of the masticatory muscles and prevents excessive force on the teeth and temporomandibular joint. Therefore, it is desirable for periodontal surgery patients with occlusion problems to consider splint treatment.

Even for patients with severe occlusion incongruity, splint treatment is very useful even when prosthetics, correction, or surgical treatment are not available.

03 Protects the occlusion adjusted by T-Scan

1 What is T-scan?

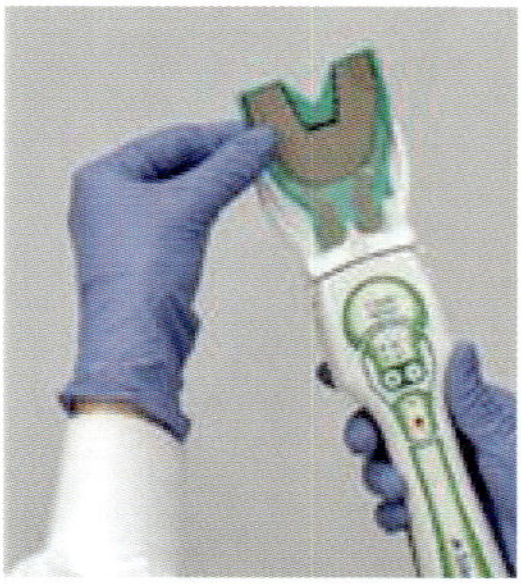

▲ Fig 34. T-scan NOVUS[4)]

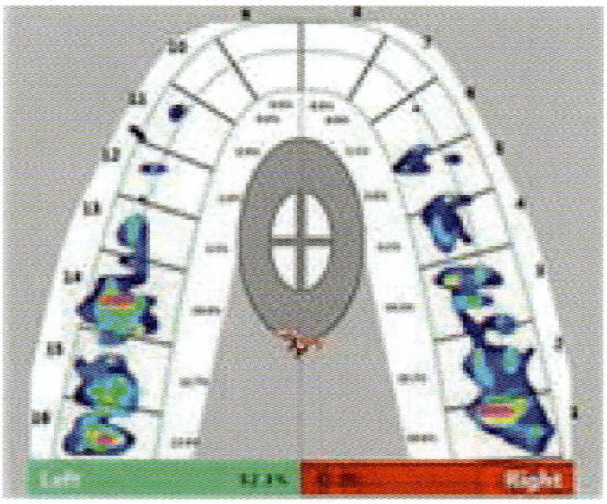

▲ Fig 35. Software view of a T-scan measurement[5)]

T-scan is a device that measures the occlusal force using a pressure sensor and saves the data as a computer graphic video over time. Abnormal occlusion can be accurately corrected to 0.1 mm. The T-scan is the only device that can accurately measure occlusal force over time. While it was developed in the 1980s by Texken in Boston, USA, it has seen a lot of improvements since then.

I personally have been using a T-scan for occlusion adjustment on all of my patients for the past 20 years. When the patient bites

4) T-scan User Manual, p.23
5) T-scan User Manual, p.33

the T-scan, the area that receives the most force over time is displayed in red, and the area that receives less force is displayed in blue on the graph.

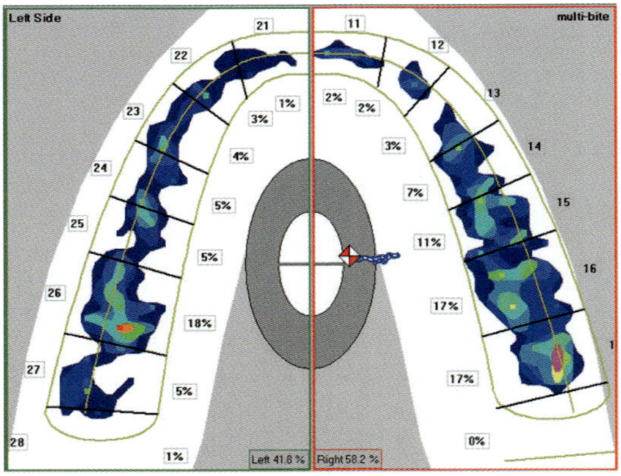

▲ Fig 36. Results of T-scan record

When the patient bites the with T-scan, the tooth area that receives the most force over time is displayed in red, and the area that receives least force is displayed in blue on the graph. During measurement, as the teeth start to occlude, the moment when one of the teeth contacts another tooth to when several teeth touch to the maximum is called the occlusal time. The goal is to reduce the occlusal time to less than 0.3 seconds so that the occlusal force is distributed to all teeth. In addition, the time when the teeth move sideways around the canines is called the disclusion time, and the goal is to reduce it to less than 0.4 seconds, so that the lateral force applied to the teeth only reaches the canines with long roots, and the other teeth are discluded. This minimizes the force exerted on the anterior and posterior teeth. Therefore, T-scan should be considered to be essential equipment for occlusion adjustment.

2 Dr. Kerstein's DTR treatment and occlusal adjustment presentation

Seminar for T-Scan users

A seminar for T-Scan users was held at Kyunghee University on February 18th and 19th, 2017. In this seminar, Dr. Robert B. Kerstein from the US presented a lecture on 'DTR (Disclusion Time Reduction) Therapy and Occlusal Adjustment'.

After the seminar, Dr. Byungkee Choi invited Dr. Kerstein to Byungkee Choi's dental office to discuss common dental occlusion concerns.

<Dental Today reported on February 24, 2017>

Dr. Robert B. Kerstein conducted a seminar on DTR (disclusion time reduction) treatment and occlusal adjustment. He emphasized that T-scan is the basis for occlusal treatment in his presentation.

After the seminar, Dr. Kerstein met with Dr. Choi Byungkee at the Byungkee Choi Dental Clinic.

On that day, Dr. Choi recalled his presentation on the correlation between occlusion and periodontal disease that he had made at the Korean Occlusal Symposium 10 years earlier. He observed how "Dr. Kerstein's DTR concept completely matches my concept that occlusal disease should be treated with occlusal adjustment."

Director Byungkee Choi continued, "I consider Dr. Kerstein's concept of using and treating with T-scan based on the DTR concept as the most efficient technology," and he emphasized, "Patients with occlusal disease should be treated with occlusal adjustment."

Director Byungkee Choi also said, "We have recommended that 5,000 patients at our hospital should wear CBK Splints, and we are also educating them on the importance of proper spine posture and abdominal breathing."

Dr. Kerstein emphasized, "There are many dentists in Korea who think that occlusal measurement is only possible with articulating paper, but for accurate occlusal measurement, you must have a T-Scan and study well so that you can use it right away."

Dr. Kerstein said, "For people with good occlusion, only the canine teeth should touch when moving the lower jaw from side to side. For accurate occlusion, DTR using T-Scan is required, and you can become the best dentist by using T-Scan effectively."

He also said, "In order to accurately diagnose occlusion, subjectivity must be excluded, but many dentists in Korea rely on the articulating paper and intuition, so it is inaccurate. It is very dangerous to do it by feeling in a situation where there is no foundation, and mistakes happen because only the size of the articulating paper is considered. Diagnosis by articulating paper is only 20~30 % reliable. Occlusal diagnosis must also consider force, and T-Scan is reliable because it can measure time and force at the same time."

This concept has been included in Korean occlusal textbooks, and the CBK Splint and anti-aging effects were explained at an International College of Prosthodontists (ICP) lecture in September 2015.

Regarding the relationship between the teeth and the whole body, "If chewing is uncomfortable, pain in the neck and back occurs, and systemic symptoms such as dizziness appear due to nutritional imbalance. Many parts of the treatment are possible by adjusting the occlusion, and since the occlusion is connected to the central nerve, relaxing the central nerve is effective for systemic symptoms."

Mr. Don Delgado (T-Scan Overseas Export Manager) said, "After people receive Dr. Kerstein's treatment, the treatment effect is so good that many of them express their gratitude by hugging him. T-Scan checks the force and time of the intersection every 3/1,000 seconds, so it is possible to check the change in force over time."

CEO Lee Won-woo (A representative of Good 'voco') also said, "According to a study by a dental team at Korea University Guro Hospital, only 35 % of dentists were checking occlusion. Like medical exams, dental exams should place importance on diagnosis, and T-Scan occupies an important position in occlusion and temporomandibular joint treatment. There are about 1,000 users in the US and about 250 users in Korea."

"This is the digital age. Dental technicians have also changed many aspects of their practice from manual work to digital using CAD/CAM, and dentists are also digitizing CT or panorama images, and recently have taken a further step with T-Scan. T-scan is not available in medical insurance, so its use should increase in the future. And it is currently available at all 11 dental college hospitals nationwide."

No matter how ideal occlusion is made with the T-Scan, teeth can be easily misaligned due to masticatory activity, bruxism, and external forces. By wearing CBK splints while sleeping, a normal occlusion can be maintained for a long time by maintaining a stable occlusion that does not become distorted.

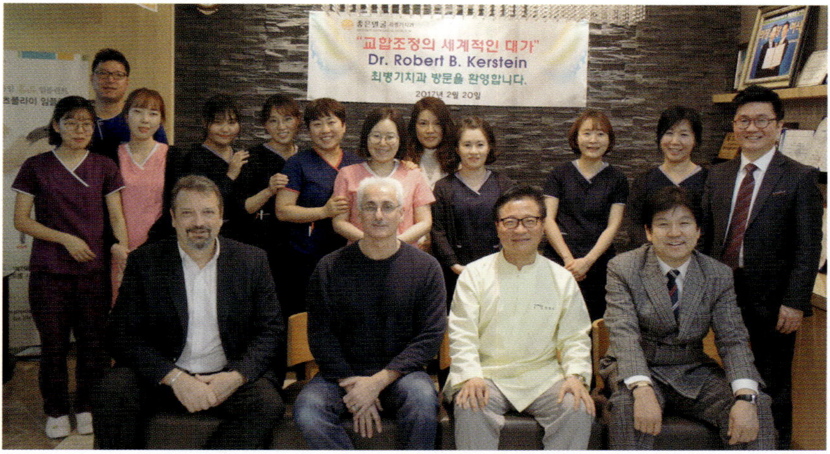
"교합조정의 세계적인 대가"
Dr. Robert B. Kerstein
최병기치과 방문을 환영합니다.
2017년 2월 20일

▲ Fig 37. (From left in the front row) Director Delgado, Dr. Kerstein, Director Byungkee Choi, and CEO Won-Woo Lee are taking a commemorative photo with Byungkee Choi's dental staff.

04 Supports a harmonious masticatory system

Dawson suggested ten conditions that constitute a harmonious masticatory system. Since these 10 elements were organically connected to each other, any problem with even one condition will affect the masticatory system.

1 Healthy temporomandibular joint

For a healthy temporomandibular joint, the following three parts must be stable.

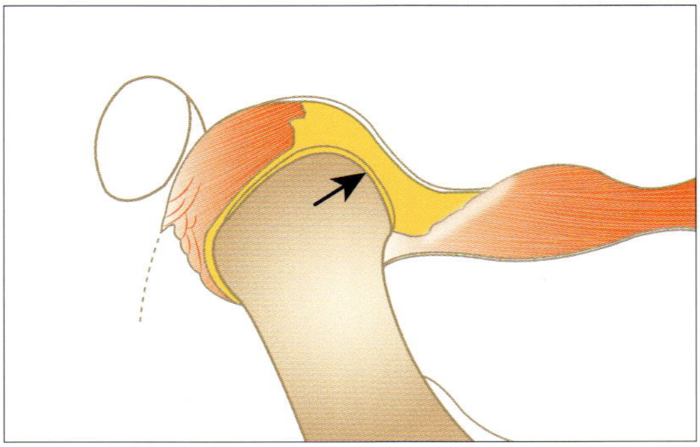

▲ Fig 38. Healthy temporomandibular joint[6)]

6) Functional Occlusion : From TMJ to Smile Design (Peter. E. Dawson, Mosby, 2006)

(1) The inferior joint cavity[7)]

This area must be stabilized as the starting point up to 25 mm where pure rotational motion of the condyle occurs when the mouth is opened.

(2) The secondary portion of the 25~50 mm aperture should be stabilized through translation from the mandibular fossa beyond the superior joint cavity articular eminence.

(3) The superior retrodiscal lamina area is very elastic and stabilizes the opening of the mouth, so this area should also be stabilized.

2 Centric Relation

The centric relation is important for a harmonious masticatory system.

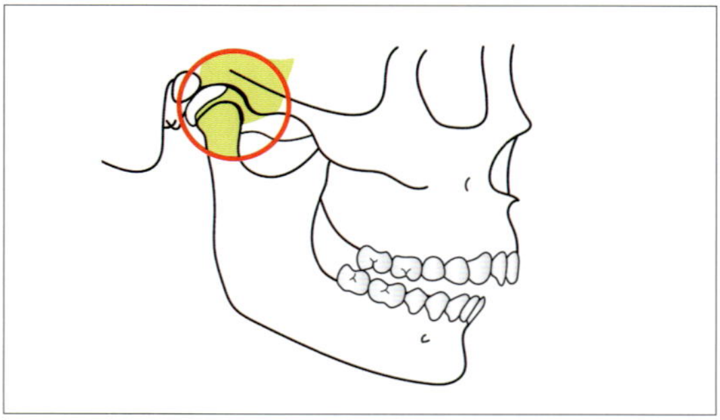

▲ Fig 39. Healthy temporomandibular joint[8)]

7) Functional Occlusion : From TMJ to Smile Design (Peter. E. Dawson, Mosby, 2006)

8) Peter. E. Dawson(2012), Functional Occlusion from TMJ to Smile Design, p.57

Two Conditions of Centric Relation

(1) When the masseter muscle, temporalis muscle, and medial pterygoid muscle contract, the physiologically stable position in which the inferior belly of the lateral pterygoid muscle relaxes is a state in which a minimum force of about 12 kg/cm^2 is received.

(2) The articular disc on the mandibular condyle must be properly positioned without falling out. Ideally, the centric relation and the maximal intercuspal position will coincide.

Brian Mill investigated 2,384 patients and announced that all patients showed differences in the centric relation and the maximal intercuspal position, so some occlusal adjustment was necessary to match them.

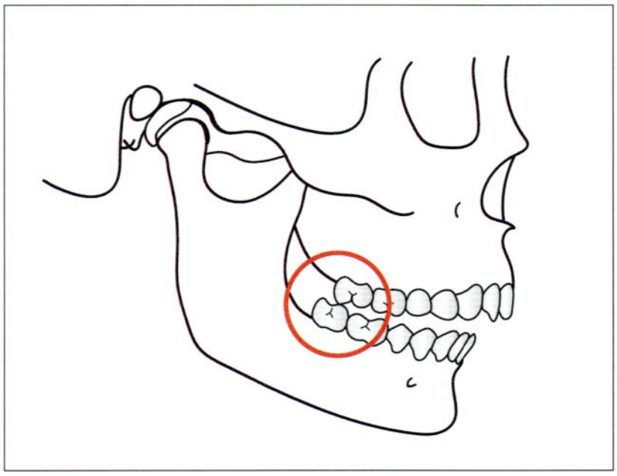

▲ Fig 40. Centric relation

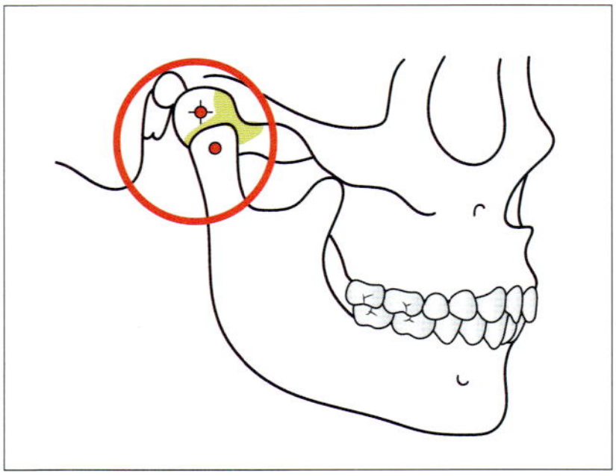

▲ Fig 41. Maximal intercuspal position

■ Ideal conditions

centric relation = maximal intercuspal position

① Occlusal adjustment ② Wearing of CBK Splint

3 The role of the masticatory muscles

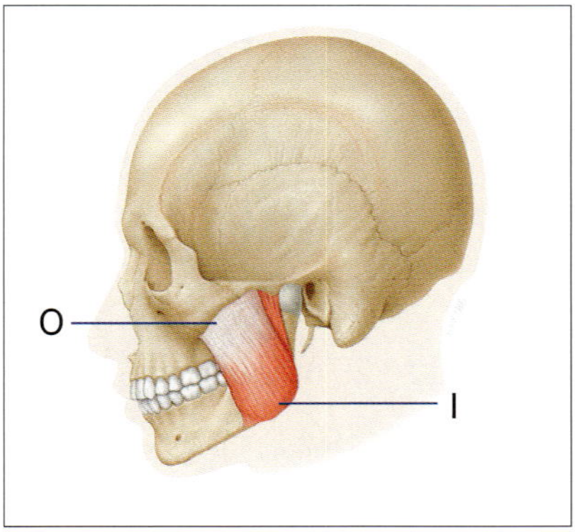

▲ Fig 42. Masseter muscle

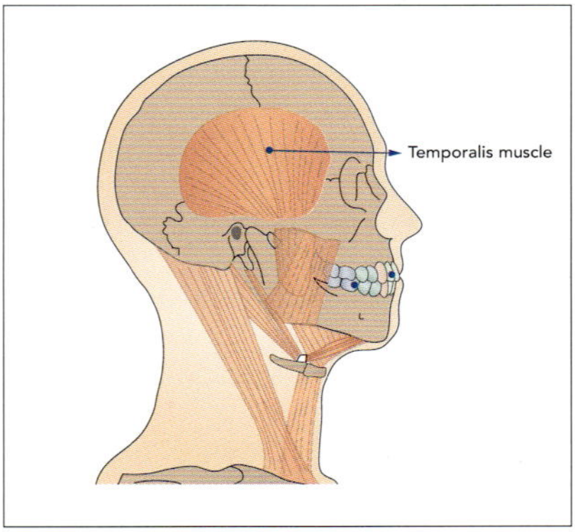

▲ Fig 43. Temporalis muscle

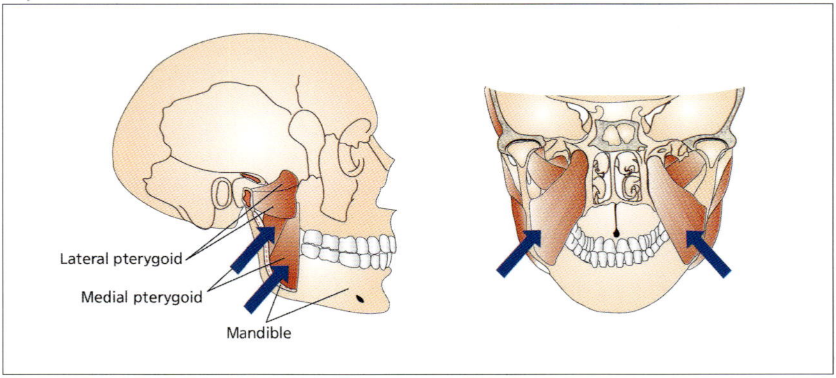

▲ Fig 44. Medial pterygoid muscle

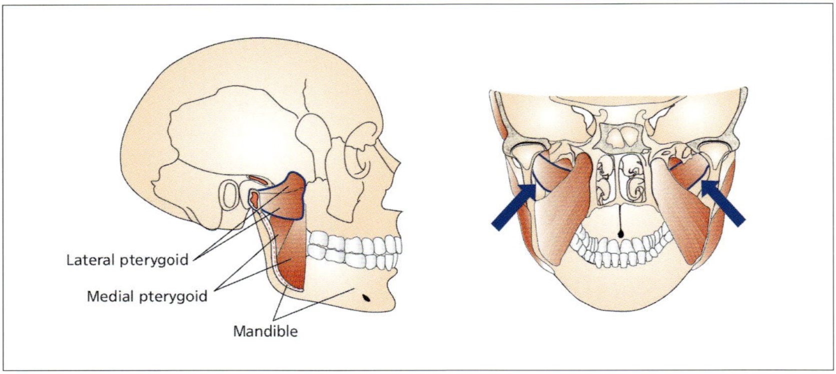

▲ Fig 45. Lateral pterygoid muscle

Physiological function (orthofuction) is an ideal state in which simultaneous occlusion occurs in the centric relation. Occlusal force is 12 ㎏/㎠ and contact occurs for 12~20 minutes a day on the cusp. Non-physiological function (parafuction, i.e., bruxism or teeth clenching) refers to a phenomenon that usually occurs during sleep or when the person is unconscious for 2~162 minutes a day with an occlusal force of 74 ㎏/㎠. This is an unphysiological muscle condition, and when this force is present, teeth crack or occlusal diseases such as attrition and cervical abrasion occur.

Furthermore, non-physiological forces can also affect the skull and the 2nd cervical vertebra, affecting overall health.

To this end, I perform occlusal adjustment and splint treatment using T-scan.

4 Anterior guidance

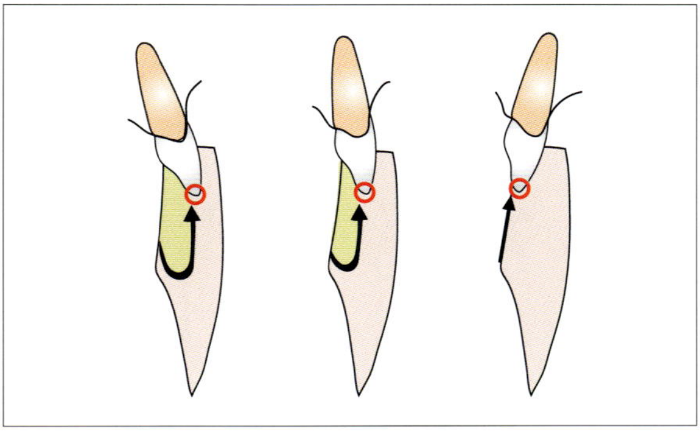

▲ Fig 46. forward movement[9)]

There should be harmonious forward movement in the anterior limit movement. If the movement of the anterior teeth is not coordinated due to occlusion when the mouth is open, a lot of occlusal force can be applied to the posterior teeth.

5 Vertical dimension

Peter Dawson says that even if the occlusion is lowered due to attrition or tooth wear, the occlusion height remains constant due to root eruption. However, when the teeth wear down, sutural jamming of the 22 cranial sutures between the skulls occurs. This

9) Peter. E. Dawson(2012), Functional Occlusion from TMJ to Smile Design, p.144

can affect the nervous system and hormones.

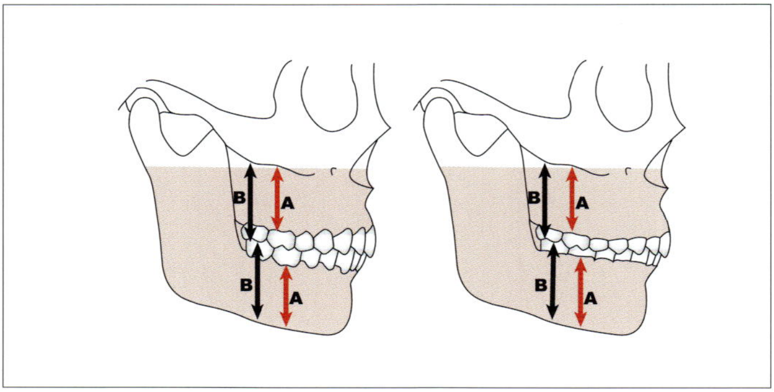

▲ Fig 47. **Vertical dimension** : The distance from the reference point of the skeleton to the occlusal surface (B) remains constant even when severe wear occurs.

6 Neutral zone

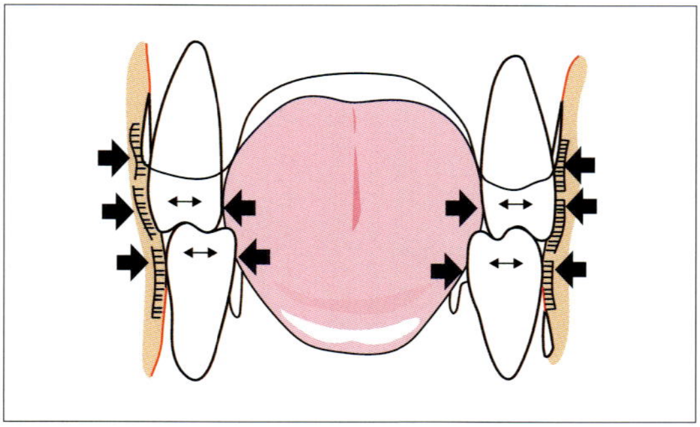

▲ Fig 48. Neutral zone[10)]

10) Peter. E. Dawson(2012), Functional Occlusion from TMJ to Smile Design, p.132, p.143, p.159

In the neutral zone, the tongue, cheeks, and teeth should be in a normal position. Everyone has a different neutral zone. Having a prosthesis outside the neutral zone will always be uncomfortable.

7 Envelope of Function

Anterior and lateral movements of the anterior teeth should be harmonious and free from jamming. If there is premature contact or occlusal interference, distortion of the masticatory muscles occurs 6~10 times more at night while sleeping, resulting in various occlusal diseases such as tooth wear, cervical abrasion, and cracked teeth.

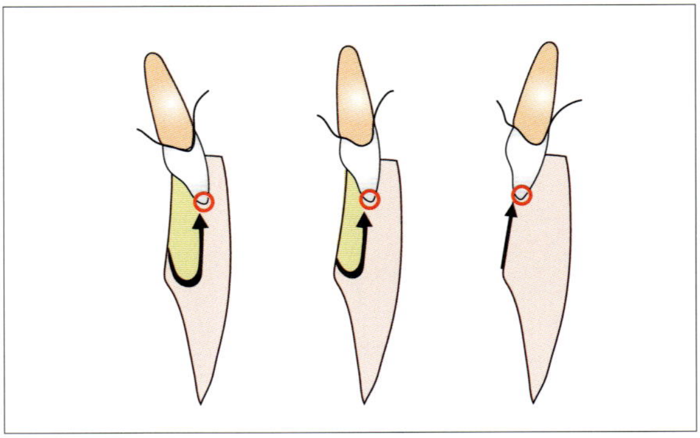

▲ Fig 49. present variations in the inclination of the upper anterior teeth.

8 Long Centric

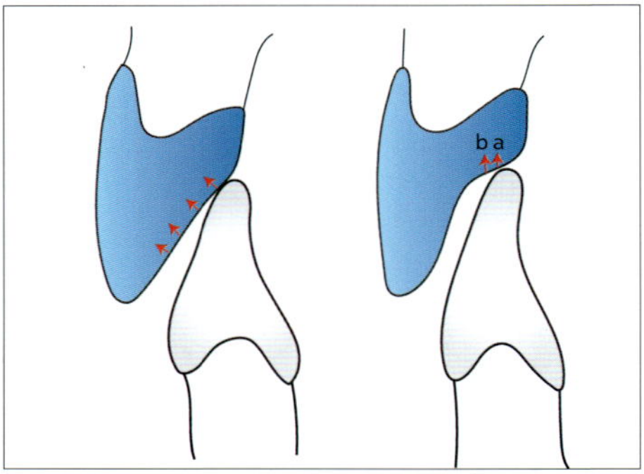

▲ Fig 50. Long centric[11)]

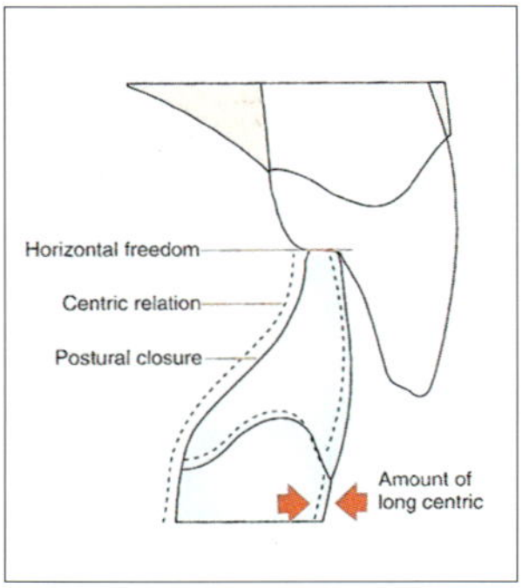

▲ Fig 51. Long centric

A space of 0.2~0.5 ㎜ is given to the lingual surface of the maxillary anterior teeth so that they can move forward and backward during forward movement.

9 Occlusal plane

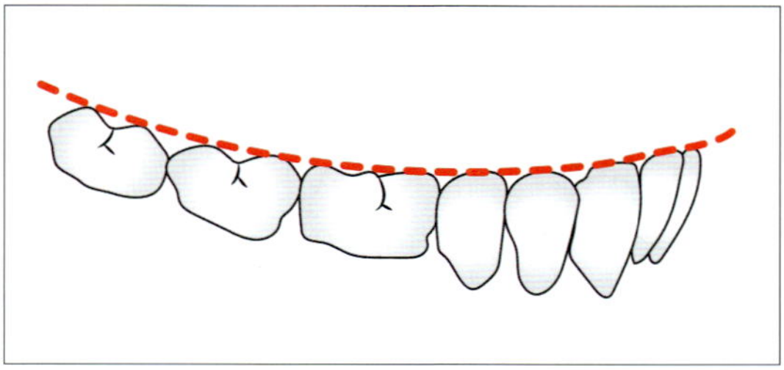

▲ Fig 52. Curve of Spee

11) Peter. E. Dawson(2012), Functional Occlusion from TMJ to Smile Design, p.140, 189

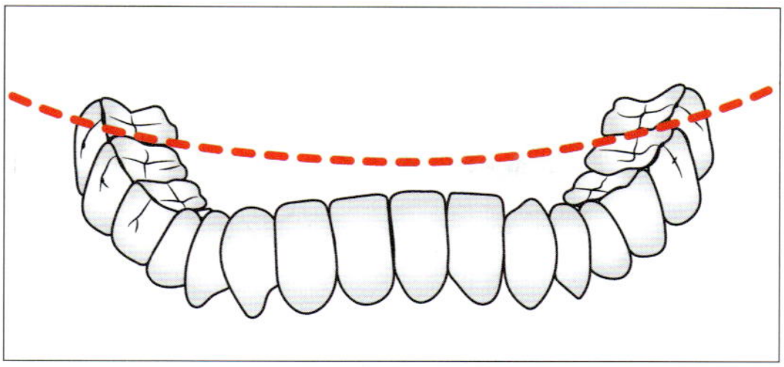

▲ Fig 53. Curve of Wilson

When the teeth are viewed from the side, there is a Curve of Spee that goes up in a circle in harmony, and when viewed from the front, there is a Curve of Wilson that harmonizes the buccal and lingual cusps. This should occur without occlusal interference during forward and lateral movements.

10 Occlusal contact plane

Harmonious anterior guidance is most important, and occlusal adjustment is performed with the concept of "Dots in back, lines in front."

The goal of occlusion treatment is to achieve simultaneous contact (maximal intercuspal position) in the centric relation. Only in this case can the masticatory muscle act with a minimum force of 12 kg/㎠, and the teeth transmit the minimum force to the skull.

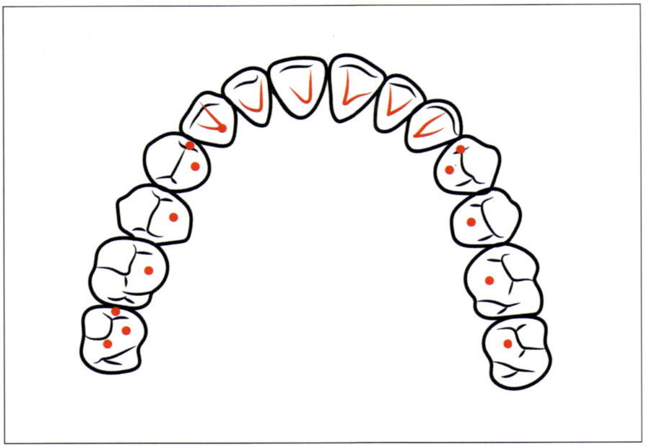

▲ Fig 54. Dots in back, lines in front.[12)]

To this end, I perform occlusion adjustment using T-scan as the first step, and if that is insufficient, I make an ideal occlusion with a CBK Splint as the second step.

12) Peter. E. Dawson(2012), Functional Occlusion from TMJ to Smile Design, p.32

05 Maintains a 'centric relation' as the key-word in dental treatment

Scholars cite 'centric relation' as the most important concept in dentistry. I also believe that the centric relation is the key to dental as well as whole- body health. Centric relation refers to a comfortable state in which the upper and lower jaws can always be reproduced regardless of occlusion.

According to Peter Dawson, the concept of centric relation is that the masseter, temporalis, and medial pterygoid muscles contract, and the inferior belly of the lateral pterygoid muscle relaxes due to antagonistic action when the temporomandibular joint is normally arranged.

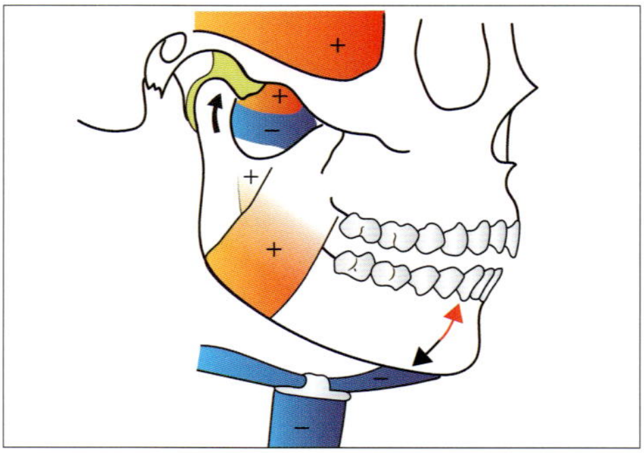

▲ Fig 55. centric relation[13)]

13) Peter. E. Dawson(2012), Functional Occlusion from TMJ to Smile Design, p.47

Coordinated muscle function refers to the appropriate relaxation of one muscle or several muscles when the antagonist muscle is contracted. When the mouth is opened, the antagonist masseter muscle contracts when the masseter relaxes. The inferior belly of the lateral pterygoid muscle contracts when the mouth is open.

There are two ways to find this important centric relation: the doctor's independent method and the patient's own method. I'll show you how to find the centric relation yourself. Let's do 'forward, backward, squeeze' using P. Dawson's movement of the mandible.

When the mandible is pulled forward and then pushed back, the first point of contact when the teeth are closed is the centric relation. In this state, the force of the facial muscles during mastication is the lowest at 12 ㎏/㎠. Also, this is the most comfortable and stable state for the skull.

When dental treatment results in one tooth being too high or the teeth do not fit, people may subconsciously masticate or just swallow when they eat during the day. However, during sleep at night, everyone performs a swallowing exercise by swallowing saliva once a minute. When this happens, 'clenching' or 'bruxism' is an unconscious compensatory action to adjust the occlusion that is high or constantly in contact.

According to R. B. Kerstein, the abnormal occlusal force at this time is 6~10 times higher than normal, that is, 72~120 kg/㎠. This force causes cervical abrasion, attrition, cracked teeth, fractures, pulpitis, periodontal disease, muscle pain, and temporomandibular joint pain. Furthermore, this force causes the masticatory muscles to distort by 6~10 times to deform the skull and temporomandibular joint as well as the spine. "It can also affect hormones and the nervous system, causing many systemic diseases," Fonder announced.

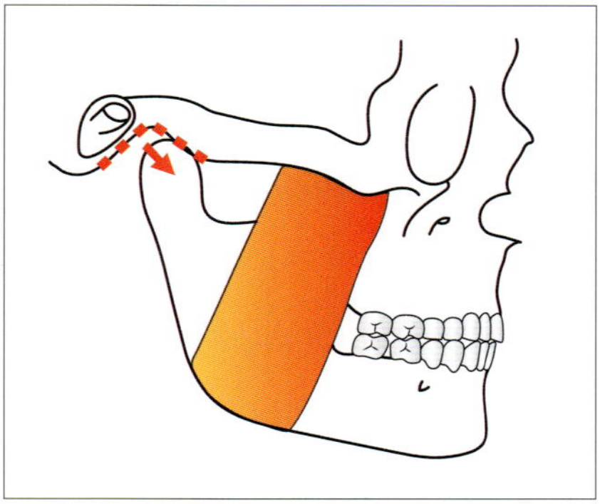

▲ Fig 56. swallowing exercise[14)]

If the condyle must move anteriorly and downward to reach the maximal intercuspal position, a mismatch between the occlusion and the temporomandibular joint will occur.

14) Peter. E. Dawson(2012), Functional Occlusion from TMJ to Smile Design, p.67

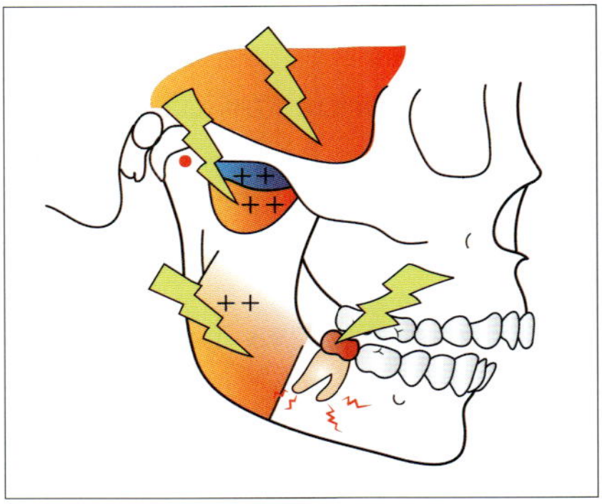

▲ Fig 57. 'clenching' or 'bruxism'[15)]

When the levator muscle pulls the condyle over the centric relation, all of the force is exerted on the posterior teeth. If the patient has clenching or bruxism during sleep, problems will arise. This is the main cause of posterior wear.

The above effects overload the posterior teeth and cause hyperactivity of the masticatory muscles. It is the most common symptom of TMD, such as occlusion, muscle, and facial pain.

In dental treatment, knowing the centric relation and achieving simultaneous occlusion (C.O. = M.I.P.) in the centric relation is the ideal occlusion, the ultimate goal of treatment pursued by masters of occlusion. In other words, if all molars are treated so that only simultaneous occlusion occurs in the centric relation and oral hygiene is well controlled by brushing teeth, the teeth are no longer damaged.

15) Peter. E. Dawson(2012), Functional Occlusion from TMJ to Smile Design, p.67

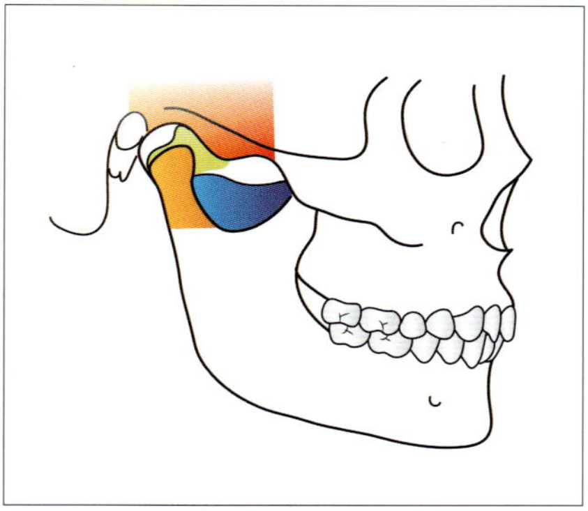

▲ Fig 58. **Type I**; When the maximal intercuspal position and centric relation are in harmony

It is extremely rare to have a practically ideal occlusion, and it is also not easy to achieve an ideal occlusion through treatment.

According to Dawson, the ideal centric relation can be created through orthodontics, prosthetics, or oral surgery.

However, these treatments can be too extensive and invasive. In response to this, I presented an alternative to create a centric relation at the 16th International College of Prosthodontists as follows.

In the first step, the occlusal force is evaluated using computer equipment called T-scan, and the occlusal adjustment is performed finely. The second step is to make simultaneous engagement in the centric relation with a CBK Splint similar to a mouthpiece.

Teeth can be easily damaged during sleep or exercise, so at these times, splints are inserted to prevent teeth from being damaged and improve the quality of sleep. Many patients who use a CBK Splint are getting good effects on immune diseases such as rhinitis and tinnitus by resolving spinal distortion or skull distortion.

Along with the CBK Splint, it is my wish that all mankind lives healthy lives with 'CBK Splint Whole-Body Health Theory' such as straightening the spine, abdominal breathing, diet control, and whole-body exercise.

06 Reduces occlusal diseases

1 Symptoms and signs

According to the medical dictionary, pain is an unpleasant sensory and emotional experience associated with actual or potential tissue damage. Pain is a symptom. People experience pain because there is tissue damage somewhere. Tissue damage is one type of sign. The sign precedes the symptom. In other words, when tissue damage occurs, pain follows. A good doctor's job is to look for what is causing the pain.

Therefore, if there is cranial pain, the doctor needs to find the cause of the pain. To this end, when the source of the pain, the cause of tissue damage (deformation), and the reason for functional dissonance are found, the doctor establishes a treatment plan.

Most importantly, the symptoms are always ongoing. It is important for the structures involved in the masticatory system to remain healthy and to be asymptomatic. Dental signs include attrition, teeth hypersensitivity, cervical abrasion, crown fissure, arthralgia, muscle pain, mouth opening disorder, and periodontal disease. When these symptoms are present, the cause must be found and treated.

2 Causes and signs of occlusal disease

In 1966, Guichet first reported pathological changes in teeth, surrounding tissues, and temporomandibular joints due to occlusal disharmony, and then in 2007, Becker published seven signs of occlusal disease of teeth due to premature contact.

They are 1) pathologic wear, 2) tooth fracture, 3) tooth hypersensitivity, 4) tooth mobility, 5) cervical abrasion, 6) gingivitis and periodontal disease, and 7) joint noise and mouth opening disorders. It was announced that periodontal disease can cause secondary loss of alveolar bone, muscle pain and temporomandibular joint pain.

Another world-renowned prosthodontist, Peter. E. Dawson announced that 'the number one cause of tooth loss today is occlusal disease, which is far more devastating than caries or periodontal disease.' Occlusal disease is caused by premature contact of one tooth because it is higher than the others and balancing interference that causes the rearmost tooth on the opposite side to deflect when chewing on just one side when eating. These phenomena cause harm to the temporomandibular joint and periodontal tissues.

3 Treatment of occlusal diseases

According to R. B. Kerstein's study, most adults with poor occlusion have 6~10 times distortion of masticatory muscles such as the masseter and temporalis. As a result, as the temporal bone and the second cervical vertebra, which are important in the human body, are distorted, nine of the 12 cranial nerves are affected, and the dura mater is distorted, affecting the hormones and the nervous system.

In order to solve this problem, occlusal adjustment is first performed through T-scan, so that the centric relation (C.R) where the upper and lower jaws are most comfortable is the centric occlusion position (C.O. = M.I.) so that multiple contact occurs. This allows mastication to happen with minimal muscle force.

After making such adjustments, a CBK Splint, Which is a kind of C.R. Splint specialized in 1.5 ㎜ thickness, should be inserted when a person is exercising or sleeping. This matches the centric relation and the maximal intercuspal position, thereby minimizing the muscle force that subconsciously occurs during swallowing movement, which is good for teeth and periodontal tissues, and allows for a deep sleep. It also has good clinical results in improving rhinitis, tinnitus, and immune diseases.

Occlusal disease treatment eliminates premature contact and occlusal interference. When treating patients, I try to create a perfect occlusal using a device called T-scan, but when that is insufficient, I use a CBK Splint.

4 Treatment of traumatic occlusion

According to the 8th prosthetics glossary in 2005, 'traumatic occlusion' refers to an occlusion that damages tissues around the teeth due to excessive functional or non-functional forces that exceed the adaptive capacity.

Traumatic occlusion occurs mainly because of premature contact where one tooth touches first, or these is occlusal interference in which contact remains too long when the tooth moves laterally, putting excessive force on the teeth or temporomandibular joint, resulting in traumatic occlusion.

The treatment of traumatic occlusion (2015 AAP) is as follows.

(1) Adjust the occlusion after examining the temporomandibular joint

(2) Advise against bad habits such as teeth clenching

(3) Stabilize agitated teeth through temporary and long-term fixation

(4) Plan orthodontic treatment

(5) Reshape the occlusion with prosthesis

(6) Stabilize occlusion by extracting specific teeth such as wisdom teeth

In the case of traumatic occlusion, I consider oral surgical treatment such as orthodontics, prosthetics, and orthognathic surgery through an overall oral examination. If these treatments are not available, the next best option is occlusal adjustment and splint treatment to form an ideal occlusion so that minimal force is applied to the masticatory muscles.

5 Classification and treatment of temporomandibular joint disease

Temporomandibular joint disease is divided into three categories:

muscle disorders, disc derangement disorders, and degenerative joint changes.

(1) Muscle disorders

When there is premature contact where a tooth touches first, pain is primarily caused in the muscles of the neck and shoulders as well as in the masticatory muscles that control the function of the temporomandibular joint. This pain is called myofascial pain, and 85 % of temporomandibular joint diseases fit into this category. Occlusal adjustment should be performed at this time.

(2) Disc derangement disorders

As the disease progresses further, the disc in the temporomandibular joint becomes dislodged, causing a sound or a disorder in which the lower jaw does not open well. If it is impossible to insert three fingers in the mouth when it is open, the occlusion should be adjusted after temporomandibular joint treatment.

(3) Degenerative disorders

When the cartilage covering the temporomandibular joint is destroyed, the temporomandibular joint is worn or torn like arthritis. Even under these conditions, occlusion adjustment should be performed after splint treatment, electric stimulation therapy, or drug therapy.

Dawson, a world-renowned prosthodontist, classified temporomandibular joint disease into four types:

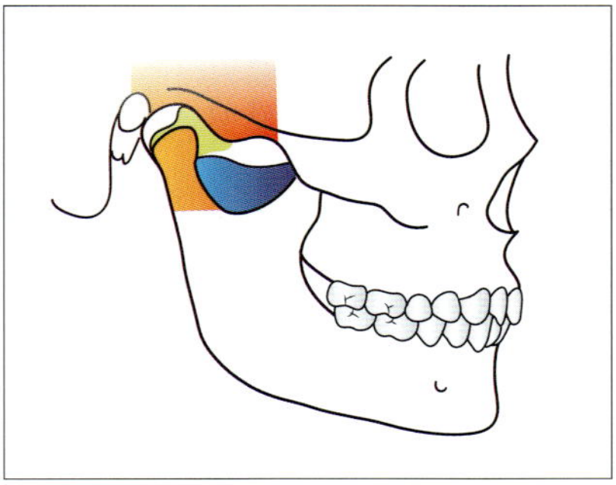

▲ Fig 59. Type 1

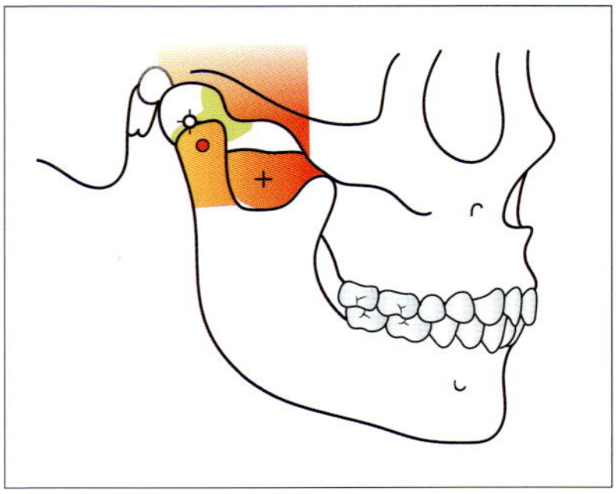

▲ Fig 60. Type 2

Type 1[16] is normal, and the articular disc, ligament and cartilage are healthy. In this state, the maximal intercuspal position occurs harmoniously in the centric relation. That is, among the masticatory muscles that affect the temporomandibular joint, the masseter muscle, temporalis muscle, and medial pterygoid muscle contract, and the inferior belly of the lateral pterygoid muscle relaxes, so that the minimum force of 12 ㎏/㎠ acts in a physiological state. When simultaneous occlusion occurs in the centric relation, that is, the maximal intercuspal position, the minimum occlusal force acts on the teeth, so that the teeth are not further damaged. The goal of treatment is to achieve this condition.

Type 2[17] is where the normal position of the joint disc is damaged due to ligament damage, fibrous atrophy of the cartilage, disc displacement, or disc perforation. In this case, the inferior belly of the lateral pterygoid muscle is distorted when biting hard (the maximal intercuspal position), and the mandibular condyle moves in the centric relation. In this condition, when there is a large difference between the centric relation and the maximal intercuspal position, or when there is occlusal interference, muscle distortion occurs about 6 times greater than normal. And at bedtime, this clenching or bruxism occurs to solve the occlusal

16) Peter. E. Dawson(2012), Functional Occlusion from TMJ to Smile Design, p.107
17) Peter. E. Dawson(2012), Functional Occlusion from TMJ to Smile Design, p.108

interference. Therefore, at this time, the centric relation should be matched with the maximal intercuspal position through occlusal adjustment, but if this is insufficient, use a CBK Splint.

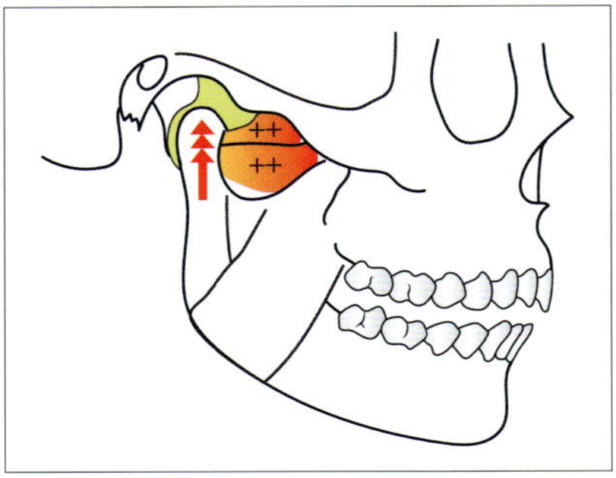

▲ Fig 61. Type 3

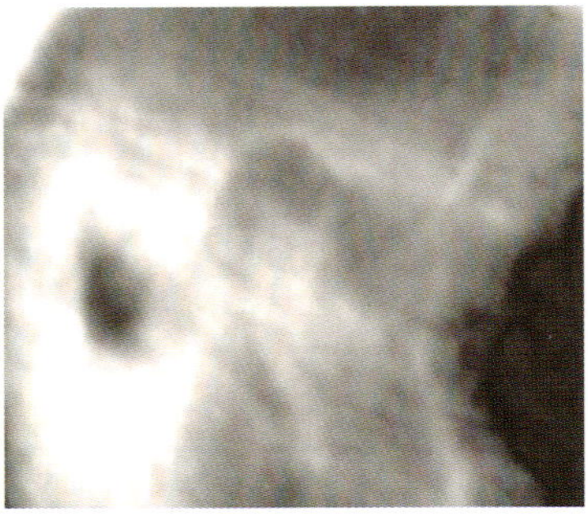

▲ Fig 62. Type 4

Type 3[18] is where the centric relation cannot be found because the joint disc is partially or completely dislocated. In this case, occlusion treatment should be performed after stabilizing the temporomandibular joint with splint treatment, physical therapy, or electrical stimulation therapy before occlusion adjustment treatment.

Type 4[19] is a degenerative change condition in which the joint disc is worn out due to a pathologically incomplete temporomandibular joint.

18) Peter. E. Dawson(2012), Functional Occlusion from TMJ to Smile Design, p.109
19) Peter. E. Dawson(2012), Functional Occlusion from TMJ to Smile Design, p.109

In summary, Type 1 is an ideal state, and Type 2 is a state of muscle imbalance, and about 85 % of temporomandibular joint patients fall into this category. Occlusal adjustment may be performed at this time. Types 3 and 4 are more advanced and account for about 15 % of patients. Splints, physical therapy, and surgical intervention are required.

07 Increases the implant success rate

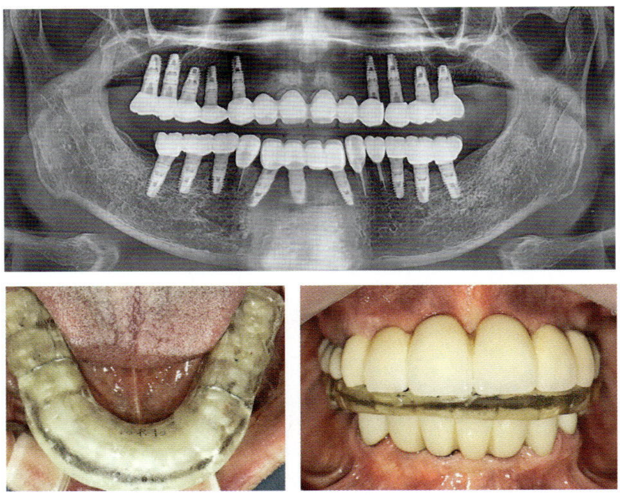

▲ Fig 63. Periodic occlusal adjustments and CBK splints are used to keep the occlusal force to a minimum in a patient with 9 maxillary and 9 mandibular implants.

Recently, implants have been in the limelight as a treatment modality after tooth extraction. They have many similarities with natural teeth in shape and function, but they have the advantage of being usable for a considerable period of time once implanted. However, implants also vary greatly depending on the patient's condition and placement method, and various problems arise if they are not managed continuously.

The biggest difference between natural teeth and implants is the presence or absence of periodontal ligament. Since natural teeth have a periodontal ligament, they can move about 56~108 ㎛ during occlusion, absorbing shock. In contrast, implants without periodontal ligament are limited to movement of 10~50 ㎛, and bone is destroyed pathologically when incorrect occlusal force is applied.

Implants have a 5~10 times greater modulus of elasticity than bone, so distortion increases during occlusal trauma, leading to destruction of the implant-bone bond.

Vertical pressure has little detrimental effect on implants. However, the harmful effect caused by horizontal force and twist is 4~5 times greater than that. Therefore, careful attention should be paid to controlling the occlusal interference after implantation.

Implants undergo pathological resorption at 60 % of the occlusal force of natural teeth. In addition, natural teeth respond to a shimstock thickness of 20 ㎛, while implants require much more detailed occlusal adjustment at 12 ㎛.

Premature contact is an important consideration with implants, but biomechanical force is more important, that is, premature contact and occlusal overload due to occlusal interference.

Under these conditions, additional implants, thicker implants (wider diameter), a narrow occlusal table, and connection between implants (splint design) should be considered to control occlusal force.

The occlusal conditions with implants are similar to those with natural teeth.

① Induce multiple simultaneous contacts from the centric relation to the posterior teeth

② Give anterior guidance that harmonizes with limit motion

③ Ideally no occlusal interference with any lateral movement

④ Promote "lips together, teeth apart"

⑤ Require CBK Splints with occlusal disease

My treatment goal is C.R.(centric relation) = M.I.(maximal intercuspal position) for all patients with occlusal disease for an ideal 12 kg/㎠ force. To this end, as a first step, a T-scan is used to reduce the occlusal time to within 0.3 seconds and the disclusion time to within 0.4 seconds for a detailed occlusal adjustment to reduce occlusal forces.

If occlusal adjustment is not sufficient, the next step is to prescribe a CBK Splint at night to minimize the harmful effects of parafunctional habits. That is, to cause C.O. = M.I.

In addition, patients are taught waist extension, abdominal breathing, and mind and environment control (exercise, diet). After treating more than 5,000 cases in this way, I have seen good improvement in not only teeth but also in whole-body health in many patients. This includes improving periodontal disease, sleep quality, and the immune system.

For square jaw patients who have developed a bruxer style due to severe distortion of the masticatory muscles, Botox injections three times every 3~4 months plus a CBK Splint help to reduce muscle strength to 60 %.

I hope to lead the world in experiencing the miracle of well-maintained teeth and implants lifelong by using occlusal adjustment and the CBK Splint that are well-preserved for indications.

08 Increases facial asymmetry treatment effects

Many people have an asymmetrical face. Facial asymmetry refers to a differences in the length or area of the left and right sides of a face, or when the slope of the lips is not parallel but is tilted to one side. It is rare for a person to have a completely symmetrical face, rather most people have a mild facial asymmetry to some degree or another.

Facial asymmetry has many causes. The method for correcting this will depend on whether the cause is due to the soft or hard tissue such as bone. Severe facial asymmetry usually requires surgery. To determine whether surgery is necessary requires a precise diagnosis based on an examination of facial bone with X-ray, a CT scan, computer analysis, tooth model production, and dental screening.

Conditions such as Romberg's disease (progressive hemifacial dwarfism) affect the soft tissue. The disease which often begins around the age of 20 causes one side of the face to become smaller, usually due to a gradual atrophy of soft tissues. It stops on its own after it has progressed for a while and can be corrected to some extent through surgery such as fat grafting or flap surgery.

Skeletal asymmetry is either congenital or it can be acquired.

When facial asymmetry is congenital, factors such as hemifacial dwarfism (craniofacial dwarfism) can be the cause. In severe cases, one ear may be small or absent, and it might be accompanied by jaw asymmetry and nerve paralysis. In comparison, acquired facial asymmetry is often caused by abnormal growth of the chin. If the jawbone or temporomandibular joint is injured at an early age, asymmetry of the jaw may develop as the child grows up.

Common characteristics of facial asymmetry include:

① Crooked eyes, nose, and mouth

② A mismatch of the center of the eyebrows and the tip of the chin or the overall centerline of the face

③ Uneven height of the corners of the mouth when smiling

④ A difference in the cheekbone positions

⑤ A mismatch in the centers of the upper and lower teeth due to a malocclusion

⑥ Food chewed with only one molar pair

⑦ A head slanted to one side

Corrective treatment methods depend on the cause of the asymmetry. When the cause is hemifacial dwarfism with bone asymmetry, treatment is complicated and takes a long time. Orthodontic surgery, bone surgery, skin and soft tissue surgery, etc. must be planned in several stages over a long period of time.

When the cause is dental malocclusion or temporomandibular joint abnormality, treatment involves correcting the centric relation through orthodontic treatment, and then wearing a CBK Splint which can increase the asymmetric treatment effect. CBK Splints are effective in correcting asymmetrical faces by relaxing the fixation of the parieto-temporal and occipito-temporal areas.

09 Protects teeth and stabilizes dentition

CBK splints are used to correct the balance of the skull by ideally adjusting the occlusion of the upper and lower jaws. In addition, they can be used to treat dental patients with various symptoms such as bruxism and snoring problems, parasympathetic nerve activation, saliva secretion promotion, and TMJ issues. The CBK Splint is similar to the regular splints, but its thickness is determined by a 1.5 ㎜ metal strip bite. The concept of intraoral treatment such as adjustment is characterized by addressing the whole-body health through systemic exercises such as spine straightening and abdominal breathing after the device is installed.

In conclusion, CBK Splints cause the maximal intercuspal position to occur simultaneously in a comfortable centric relation of the temporomandibular joint, and the induced anterior contact to occur when the mandible is pushed forward. With the CBK Splint, it is possible for people to keep their teeth for life and to enjoy the comfortable effect they have on the skull.

After teeth have been adjusted to the ideal occlusion, there will be no deformation of the teeth, gingiva, and temporomandibular joint. This means CBK Splints help to maintain ideal conditions after orthodontic treatment or facial asymmetry treatment.

chapter 04

CBK Splints and Whole-body Health

01 Upright spines and improved health

02 Stabilizes cerebrospinal fluid flow

03 Correct occlusion stabilizes the nervous system

04 Correct occlusion stabilizes the endocrine (hormone) system

05 Five components of Whole-body Health

01 Upright spines and improved health

1 The importance of spine posture

The spine is the key that holds our bodies upright. Whole-body health can be maintained when the skull, spine, and pelvis are connected and organically functioning together. Therefore, aligning the spine correctly is necessary to improve the health of the whole body. In the 1900's, D.D. Palmer famously said, "When the spine is upright, the Innate Intelligence (the immune system) works." In addition, Tinbergen, who won the Nobel Prize in 1973, announced that "Alexander Normalization," that is, correcting bad posture in the human body, reduces mental and physical diseases. If the posture of the spine is not right, the human body is discordant in three parts of the skull, spine, and pelvis.

The spine is comprised of 24 bones. There are 7 cervical vertebrae, 12 thoracic vertebrae, and 5 lumbar vertebrae. The most important of these vertebrae is the 2nd cervical vertebrae (axis). Further, there are about 600 muscles in the human body, and among them, 138 pairs of muscles are directly or indirectly connected to the axis.

When the axis (C2) is distorted, the atlas (C1) becomes

immediately distorted, and the rest of the spine is distorted as a domino effect, and the pelvis and skull are distorted as well. Therefore, the axis plays the most important role in the balance of the spine.

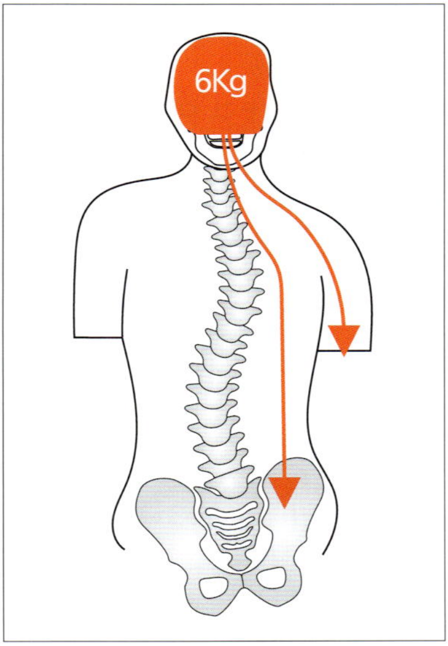

▲ Fig 64. Crooked spine and pelvis

While the axis is important, the temporomandibular joint is also important because it is deeply related to the spine. The causes of imbalance in the temporomandibular joint are malocclusion, unilateral chewing habits, missing teeth, head and neck trauma, bad posture, hard food, and chewing a lot of gum. Additionally, trauma, stress, and imbalance of the temporomandibular joint can distort the cranial sutures and affect the rhythm of the skull's movement. Eventually, it can disrupt the flow of cerebrospinal fluid and affect the central nervous system.

Therefore, the temporal bone and 2nd cervical vertebrae (axis) are the most important things in the balance of the skull and spine, and these two bones are directly affected by the occlusion of the teeth.

When the skull is in the correct position, approximately 6 ㎏ of weight is placed on the spine, but when the head is bent forward or sideways, about 20 ㎏ of weight is applied to the spine. Therefore, posture with an upright head is good for the spine.

2 Spine and tooth occlusion

If the teeth are misaligned, the masseter, temporalis, medial pterygoid, and lateral pterygoid muscles receive 6~10 times the wrong force. This force is applied towards the origin of the muscles can distort the cranial sutures. As a result, it can affect hormones and the nervous system and cause various kinds of diseases.

In addition, when the spine is leaning or is not in the right posture, it causes spinal diseases such as spinal stenosis, spinal curvature. As such, spinal diseases are closely related to incorrect posture and bad occlusion.

Even if the pelvis is twisted, the spine and skull are affected together. In 1984, American dentist G.H. Smith also announced that various problems (skull, temporomandibular joint, pelvic, nutritional, muscular, organ, and mental problems) cause interrelated diseases. Among them, posture and occlusion have the greatest influence on the skull, temporomandibular joint, and pelvis.

The spine is made up of 24 bones. All organs are connected to the spine as shown in <Fig 65, 66>.

If the spine is not in the correct posture or the occlusion is abnormal, the facial muscles can be distorted by 6~10 times more than normal, and the temporomandibular joint becomes distorted, which causes the spine to be distorted. When the spine is distorted by the skull, the function of each organ can be reduced by 20~30 %.

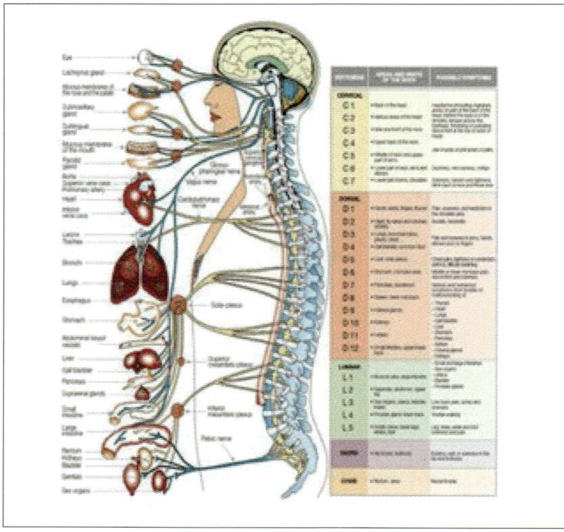

▲ Fig 65. A schematic diagram of the organic relationship between each organ and the spine

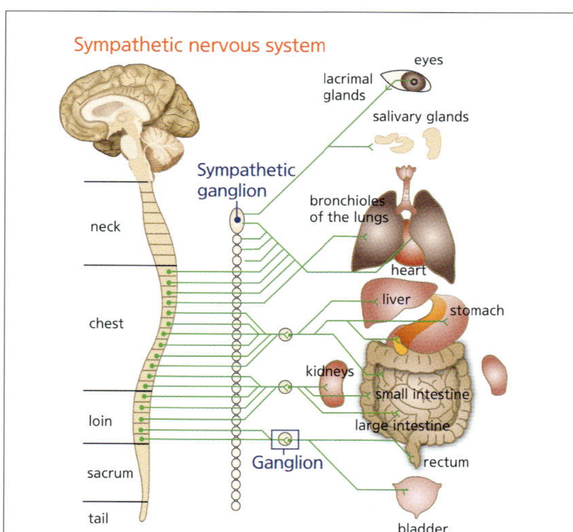

▲ Fig 66. Organs connected to the spine

The importance of proper posture was highlighted in the 1900s when Palmer published his famous statement, "The spine in good posture activates the immune system." Also in 1973, Tinbergen won the Nobel Prize for announcing that many mental and physical diseases are cured by correcting wrong postures.

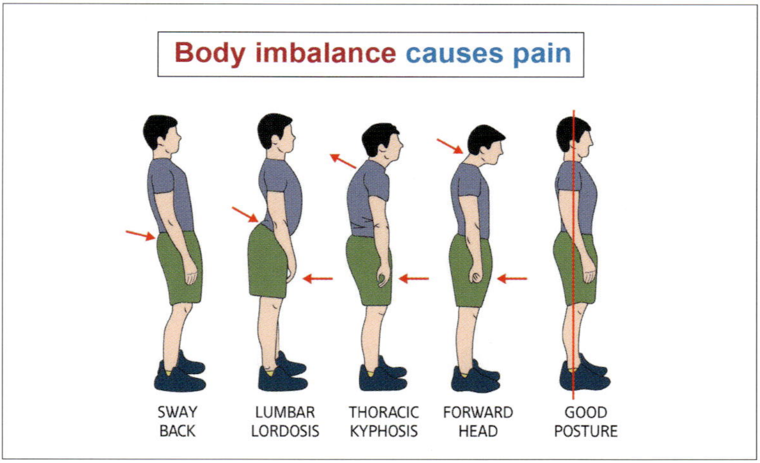

▲ Fig 67. Various postures of the spine[20)]

The correct spine posture is shown in <Fig 67>. For good spine posture, it is important to never lean on anything else and support the spine with your own muscles. This is because, as the saying goes, "Bones cannot beat muscles." Bones and teeth are controlled by muscles. Therefore, it is always wise to consciously stretch your back muscles and maintain good posture.

20) https://m.blog.naver.com/ajacademy/150181767600

Gait is also important <Fig 68>. I am convinced that if these things were to be practiced well, the national public health would improve by 20~30 %, so patients who visit our hospital are always educated and encouraged to practice good posture.

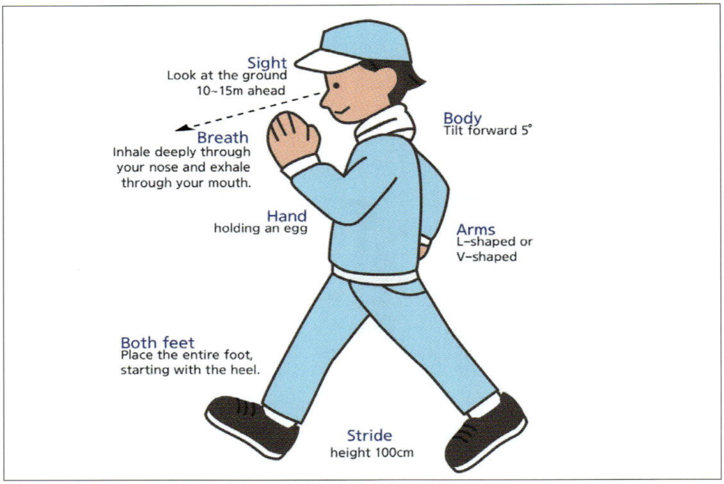

Sight
Look at the ground 10~15m ahead
Breath
Inhale deeply through your nose and exhale through your mouth.
Hand
holding an egg
Body
Tilt forward 5°
Arms
L-shaped or V-shaped
Both feet
Place the entire foot, starting with the heel.
Stride
height 100cm

▲ Fig 68. Correct Walking Posture

3 Straighten the spine by adjusting tooth occlusion

Along with correct posture, dental occlusion has a great influence on the spine. Let's learn how occlusion of teeth affects the health of the whole body.

If you neglect a missing tooth, have a habit of chewing on only one side when eating, or if your teeth are not in harmony, the four large chewing muscles (masseter, temporal, medial pterygoid, and lateral pterygoid muscles) in the maxillofacial area receive force 6~10 times higher than normal.

These abnormal forces can be controlled during the day by being aware of them, but at night or in an unconscious state, a compensatory action occurs to adjust the occlusion that can have negative consequences.

As a result, attrition, cracked teeth, periodontal disease, muscle pain, and temporomandibular joint pain may occur. Temporomandibular joint displacement <Fig 69> causes masticatory pain and is one of the most predictable and treatable causes.

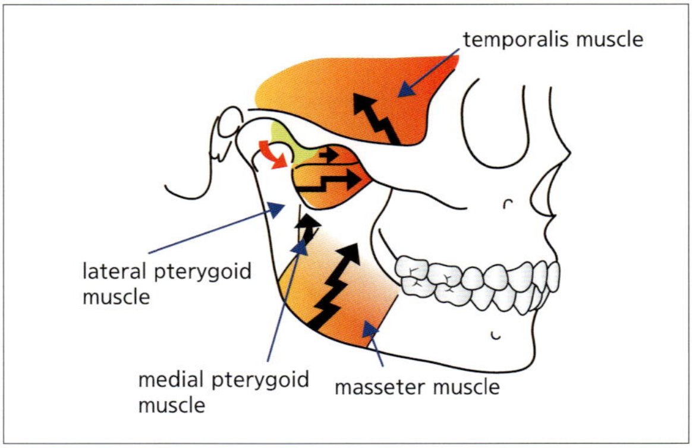

▲ Fig 69. Temporomandibular joint displacement[21)]

21) Peter. E. Dawson(2012), Functional Occlusion from TMJ to Smile Design, p.49

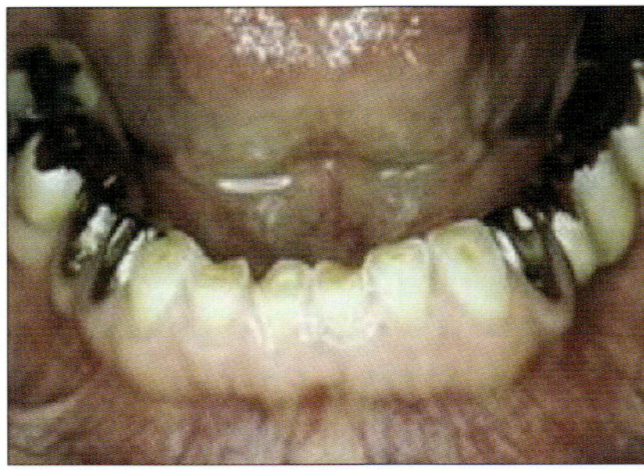

▲ Fig 70. Muscles react to eliminate tooth surface collisions caused by bruxism or nonfunctional friction.

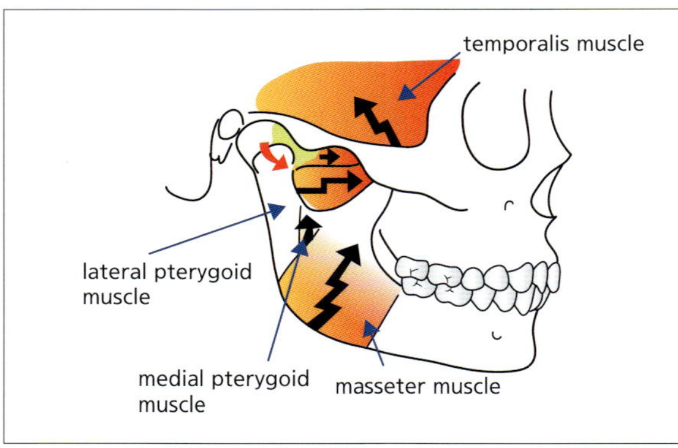

▲ Fig 71. Masticatory muscle pain[22)]

Occlusal disorders can potentially cause masticatory muscle pain <Fig 70>. The position of the temporomandibular joint changes to facilitate occlusion at the maximum intercuspal position, and this is the cause of the greatest pain in the masticatory muscles <Fig 71>.

In addition, looking at the whole body, the skull is composed of 22 bones, and each bone is composed of sutures having a gap of

22) Peter. E. Dawson(2012), Functional Occlusion from TMJ to Smile Design, p.25

about 250 microns. However, when abnormal forces are applied, the gap between sutures narrows, reducing the movement of the temporal bone, which plays an important role in overall health.

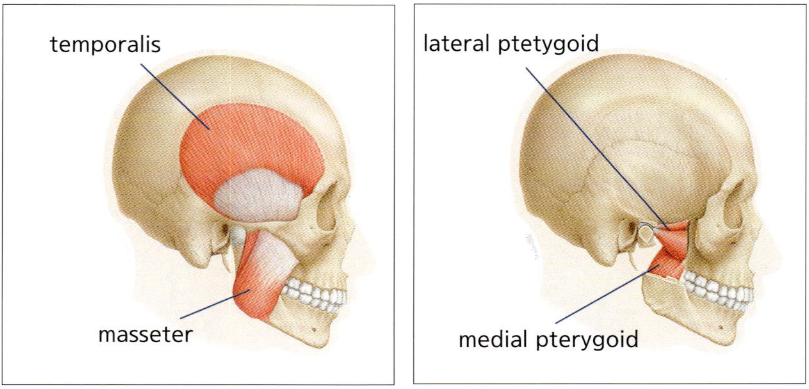

▲ Fig 72. 4 large masticatory muscles

According to C. M. Guzay's Quadrant Theory (1979), the aforementioned forces distort the first (atlas) cervical and second (axis) cervical vertebrae. Distortion of the 2nd cervical vertebra affects 24 vertebrae, potentially distorting all vertebrae.

According to Fonder, another scholar, trauma or temporomandibular joint dissonance distorts the skull, hinders the flow of cerebrospinal fluid, and distorts the shape of the skull itself, affecting the central and peripheral nerves.

Of the 12 cranial nerves, 9 affect the temporomandibular joint. In particular, the 5th nerve (trigeminal nerve) is connected to the axis, and 136 muscles are directly or indirectly connected to the axis, which affects the health of the whole body.

Our body is connected by over 600 muscles. However, among the them, 272 muscles are connected to the temporomandibular joint, so when tooth occlusion is misaligned, it affects the temporomandibular joint, temporal bone, and cervical spine <Fig 73>.

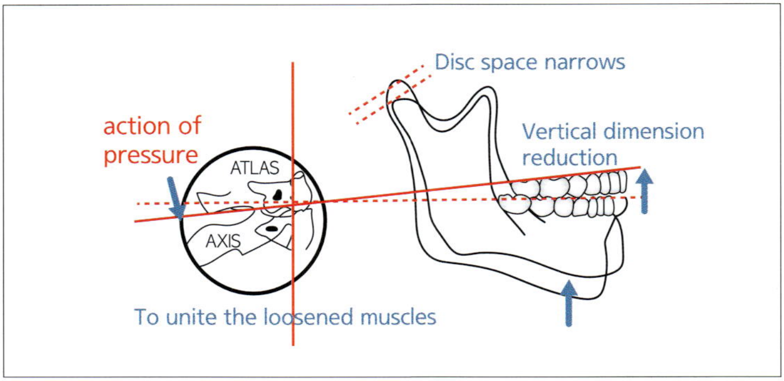

▲ Fig 73. TMJ imbalance puts pressure on the cervical spine.

When the temporomandibular joint is imbalanced, the wear and tear caused by misalignment of the teeth lowers the occlusal height and narrows the disc space of the temporomandibular joint. In addition, due to these phenomena, compression force can be applied to the first and second cervical vertebrae and muscles can become sore.

On the other hand, if dental treatment or splints (occlusion stabilizers) increase the vertical dimension and balance the temporomandibular joint, the space of the temporomandibular joint disc widens and acts as a traction force on the cervical vertebrae <Fig 74>, loosening the sore muscles associated with the 1st and 2nd cervical vertebrae <Fig 75>.

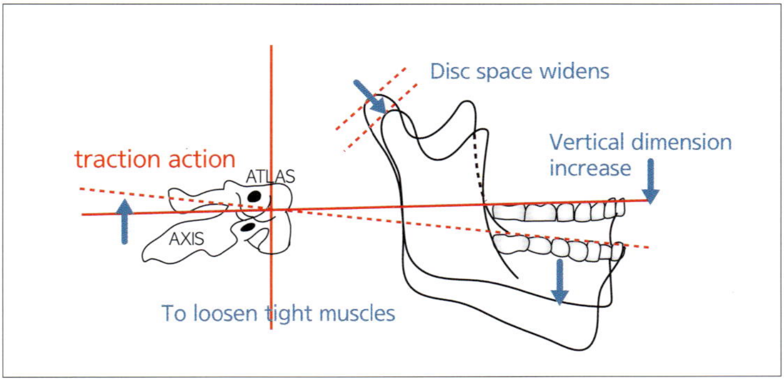

▲ Fig 74. TMJ balance acts on traction on the cervical vertebrae to stabilize the disc, occlusal height, and muscles.

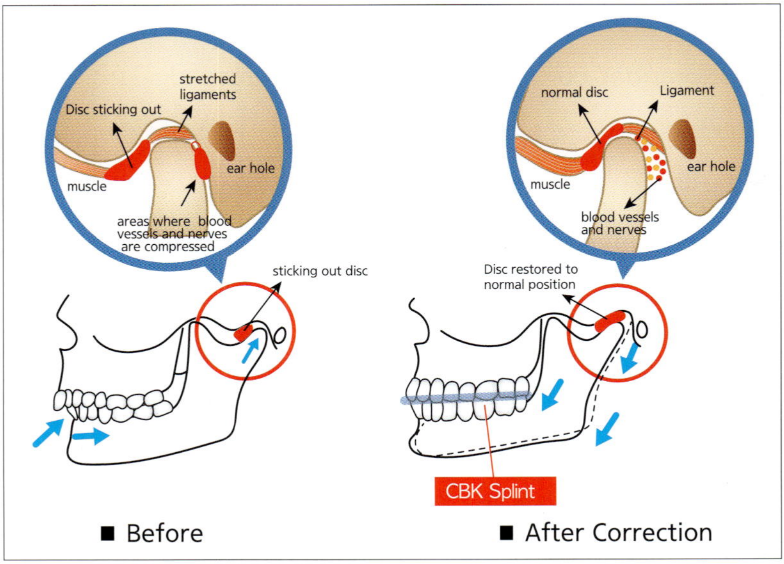

▲ Fig 75. Schematic diagram before and after treatment of temporomandibular joint disorder

4 CBK Splint effects to straighten the spine

In September 2015, at the International College of Prosthodontists (ICP) Conference, I lectured on the theory of CBK Splint Whole-Body Health. At that conference, it was announced that if the spine is erected correctly, adults with misaligned occlusion wear the CBK Splint when sleeping or exercising, and practice abdominal breathing, eat a balanced diet, and exercise regularly, their whole-body health will be improved.

More than 5,000 patients in my hospital have worn CBK Splints while sleeping for a correct posture of the spine, which has the effect of preventing distortion of the skull caused by distortion of the masticatory muscles. In addition, abdominal breathing, meditation, diet control, and exercise improve diseases caused by structural abnormalities or diseases related to immunity. With a similar effect, sometimes patients with missing teeth or a very low vertical dimension can see a remarkably improved complexion and health when vertical dimension is increased with prosthetics, implants, or dentures. Therefore, it can be seen that occlusion has a great effect on the overall health of our bodies.

Recently, I heard about a dental clinic that cares about general health and treats patients through collaboration with an internal medicine doctor. The fact that a dentist treats in collaboration with other doctors is in line with the author's idea that "the human body is organically connected, and the spine is at the center of the human body, so dental occlusion plays an important role in the health of the whole body." I think it's a very proper thing to do.

02 Stabilizes cerebrospinal fluid flow

1 Effects of malocclusion on the skull -Cranial Rhythmic Impulse (CRI) and Health-

The skull has a rhythmic impulse (beat) of 10~14 times a minute apart from breathing. Whenever the skull breathes, the sphenoid and occipital bones flex and elongate <Fig 76>. In addition, with every breath, the temporal bone rotates inward and outward. This represents the flow of cerebrospinal fluid. For example, when someone is in a coma, the rhythmic impulse (CRI) is reduced to 3 or 4 times per minute.

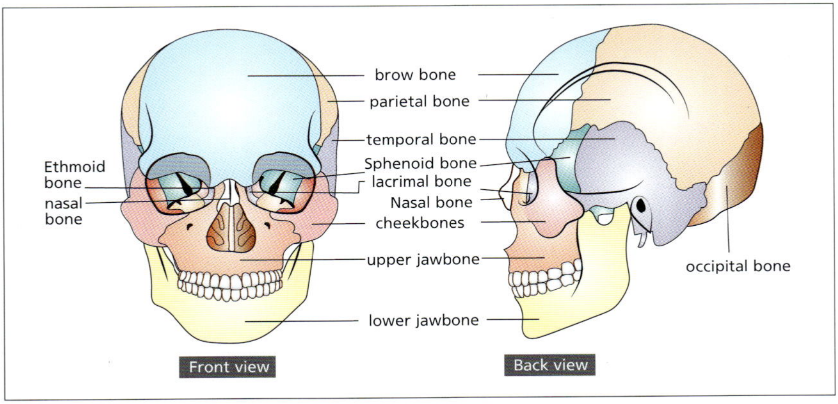

▲ Fig 76. Bones and sutures in the skull

As we age, premature contact or occlusal interference in which the teeth continue to touch occurs, resulting in chronic occlusal incongruity. In order to solve the malocclusion while sleeping, the four masticatory muscles (masseter, temporal, medial pterygoid, lateral pterygoid muscles) become distorted due to unconscious clenching and bruxism.

The occlusal force, (originally 12 ㎏/㎠ in the physiological centric relation) which is applied to the masticatory muscles in the case of malocclusion, is 74~100 ㎏/㎠. In this case, attrition, cervical abrasion, cracked teeth, and tooth hypersensitivity can occur along with abnormal muscles of the temporomandibular joint and disc deformation of the temporomandibular joint.

This same distortion also affects the skull. The skull is held together by 22 bone fragments. However, when a strong distorted force is applied due to malocclusion, suture jamming of the temporal parietal bone and the occipital temporal bone occurs. With this sutural jamming, the normal 250 ㎛ of sutural movement is reduced and the internal and external rotation of the temporal bone is restricted. According to C.M.Guzay's quadrant theory, the muscles connected around the 1st (atlas) and 2nd (axis) cervical vertebrae become distorted, and as a result, the Lovett brother's reaction causes disharmony of the entire spine.

In addition, the cranial rhythmic impulse (CRI) of the skull is discordant, and the dura mater is distorted, obstructing the flow of cerebrospinal fluid. These reactions affect the nervous system and hormones, which can cause various diseases.

2 Malocclusion and obstruction of cerebrospinal fluid flow (CSF)

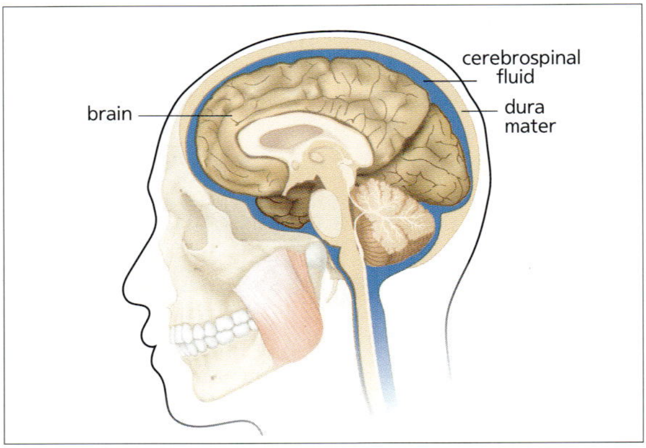

▲ Fig 77. Cerebrospinal fluid in the brain

About 500 ㎖ of Cerebrospinal Fluid (CSF) is produced in the Choroid Plexus inside the ventricle <Fig 77>. Cerebrospinal fluid is a clear, colorless fluid that circulates through the brain and spinal cord along the subarachnoid space. It is decomposed and absorbed in the arachnoid granules by 100 to 150 ㎖ every 4~6 hours.

The central nervous system, such as the brain and spinal cord, is surrounded by meninges and supported by colorless and transparent cerebrospinal fluid to exist floating in space. The brain weighs about 1,400 g, but buoyancy due to the cerebrospinal fluid, makes it effectively only 50 g, so the brain can maintain its shape without being crushed.

Cerebrospinal fluid protects the brain and spinal cord from the external environment and shock. It also transports hormones to the brain, regulates electrolytes, and maintains homeostasis which sustains brain function.

In addition, a recent Boston University research team published in the Science Journal that "cerebrospinal fluid plays a role in discharging waste products during sleep." It was found that this cerebrospinal fluid flows according to the cranial rhythmic impulse of brain waves (CRI) and it was confirmed that toxic proteins generated in the brain were removed. If this protein is not excreted and accumulates, it interferes with the flow of information in the brain. Furthermore, the accumulation of beta amyloid causes Alzheimer's disease. "With age, the cranial rhythmic impulse (CRI) decreases, which leads to a decrease in blood flow to the brain and cerebrospinal fluid the whole body.," it was announced.

Malocclusion of the teeth causes disharmony in the cranial rhythmic impulse (CRI) of the skull, and the dura matter is distorted, which hinders the flow of cerebrospinal fluid. This adversely affects the health of I believe that correct spinal posture, ideal occlusion, and abdominal breathing are important to structurally facilitate the flow of cerebrospinal fluid.

03 Correct occlusion stabilizes the nervous system

The nervous system is largely divided into the central nervous system, which consists of the brain and spinal cord, and the peripheral nervous system, which consists of the somatic and autonomic nerves <Fig 78>.

The central nervous system is the network that synthesizes incoming stimuli and produces a response. The peripheral nervous system is in the form of nerve fibers and plays a role in transmitting stimuli and responses to sensory organs, muscles, and internal organs in the form of electrical signals.

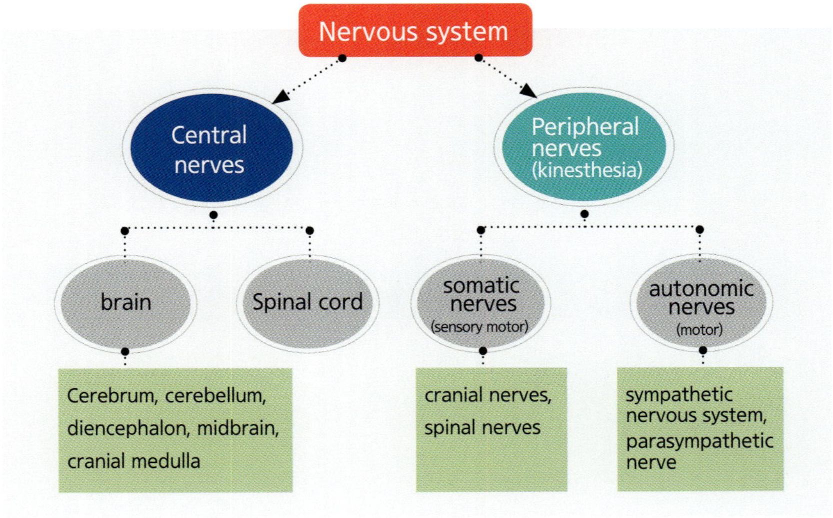

▲ Fig 78. Nervous system

The central nervous system mainly consists of associated neurons. The peripheral nervous system consists of sensory neurons that receive stimuli and transmit them to the central nervous system, and motor neurons that transmit responses made in the central nervous system to all parts of the body.

The central nervous system can also be divided into the somatic nervous system, which can be controlled consciously, and the autonomic nervous system, which cannot be consciously controlled. The autonomic nervous system is divided into the sympathetic nervous system and the parasympathetic nervous system, which mainly antagonize each other.

Correct posture, dental occlusion, and abdominal breathing can affect the central nervous system, which consists of the brain and spine.

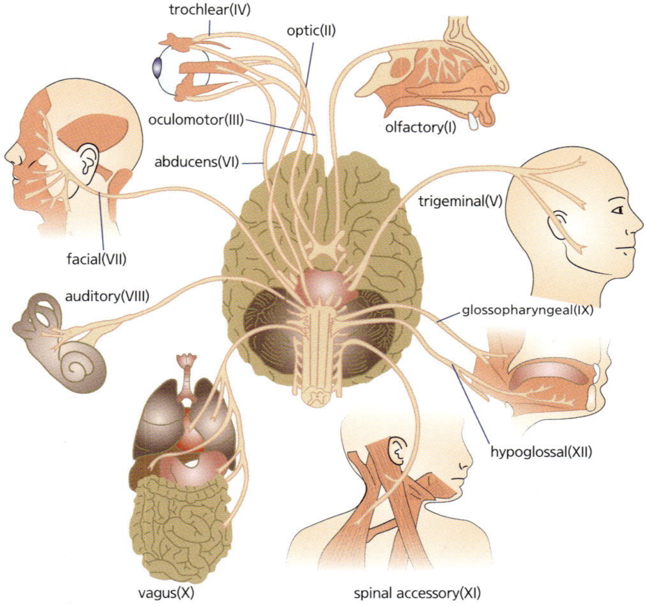

▲ Fig 79. 12 Pairs of Cranial Nerves[23)]

The somatic nervous system consists of 12 pairs of cranial nerves and 31 pairs of spinal nerves <Fig 79>. Sutural jamming of the cranial sutures due to incorrect posture of the brain or spine or malocclusion of the teeth can affect the activities of the central nervous system and the peripheral nervous system.

23) https://ko.m.wikipedia.org/wiki/%ED%8C%8C%EC%9D%BC:%EB%87%8C%EC%8B%A0%EA%B2%BD_12%EA%B0%9C%EC%9D%98_%EB%AA%A8%EC%8B%9D%EB%8F%84_%EA%B5%AC%EC%A1%B0.jpg)

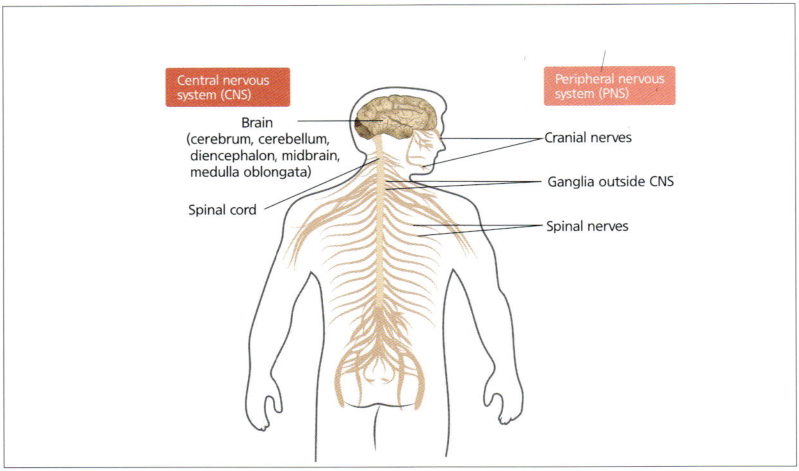

▲ Fig 80. Nerous System

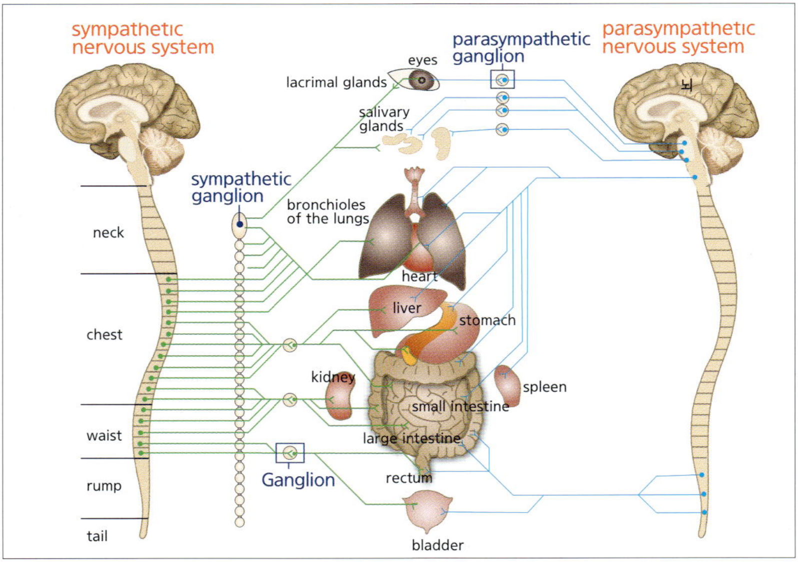

▲ Fig 81. Nervous system

The autonomic nervous system is divided into the sympathetic nervous system and the parasympathetic nervous system <Fig 80> and plays an essential role in vital activities such as digestion, heartbeat, and secretion of hormones. This happens unconsciously and without cerebral influence. Noradrenaline is secreted at the end of the sympathetic nervous system and acetylcholine is secreted at the end of the parasympathetic nervous system. They antagonize each other to control the internal organs <Fig 81>.

The sympathetic nervous system acts on the thoracic and lumbar vertebrae in a "fight-or-flight response" and becomes active when the body moves a lot or when stress increases in a fearful situation. Conversely, in a relaxed state, the parasympathetic nervous system is activated. The parasympathetic nervous system is a 'digest and rest response.' The parasympathetic nerve is associated with the 3rd cranial nerve (oculomotor), 7th cranial nerve (facial), 9th cranial nerve (glossopharyngeal), and 10th cranial nerve (vague) and vertebrae 1 and 2.

According to Fonder, if the occlusion of the teeth is misaligned, the temporomandibular joint is distorted, which causes the cervical number 2 (axis) to be distorted and immediately causes the cervical number 1 (atlas) to be distorted. Also, because of this distortion, 9 of the 12 cranial nerves, (excluding the 1st, 2nd, and 12th nerves) are said to be affected. In particular, the 10th cranial nerve (the vague nerve) is affected, which greatly affects many organs such as the lungs, digestive system, and liver. In this way, dental malocclusion causes disorders of the peripheral nervous system. In addition, an abnormal temporomandibular joint directly stimulates the trigeminal nerve and puts pressure on the nerve roots of the first and second cervical vertebrae.

It was announced that this can cause many diseases related to the central nervous system by directly stimulating the central nervous system. Occlusal disharmony has a negative effect on the cranial rhythmic impulse (CRI) of the skull and adversely affects the nervous system, resulting in various diseases.

If occlusion is increased or a patient whose skull has been distorted due to the damage caused by poor occlusion wears a CBK Splint, it has the effect of improving the periodontal disease, improving the quality of sleep, and improving digestion, as well as comforting the mind and activating the parasympathetic nervous system.

04 Correct occlusion stabilizes the endocrine (hormone) system

The human body is controlled and regulated by the nervous and endocrine systems.

The nervous system works through neurons when you do something quick and direct, like picking up a cup of coffee or kicking a soccer ball. On the other hand, the endocrine system works in a very wide range of actions, such as slowing blood flow by secreting hormones or binding to receptors in several different organs. The nervous system enables complex and sophisticated movements to be performed harmoniously, while the endocrine system regulates various physiological phenomena and behaviors. The body needs hormone secretion to regulate emotions such as stress, sleep, sadness, and joy.

The pituitary gland under the hypothalamus is the main gland that controls all hormones. Ninety-five percent of all hormones are regulated by the hypothalamus. The nervous system and hormones also work to maintain the homeostasis of body temperature, blood sugar, and water content. Hormones secreted by the pituitary gland can activate other endocrine gland cells, such as adrenal stimulating hormones and thyroid stimulating hormones. In addition, it can greatly affect physiological functions of the body, such as body temperature, circadian rhythm, hunger, and sleep.

Thyroid hormone is involved in body temperature regulation and energy metabolism, and the parathyroid gland controls calcium concentration. The adrenal gland secretes adrenaline and epinephrine, which respond to stress, regulate the immune response, constrict blood vessels, and regulate blood pressure. Alpha cells in the pancreas secrete insulin, which lowers blood sugar. Beta cells secrete glucagon, which increases blood sugar. The ovaries in women secrete the female hormone estrogen, and the testes in men secrete the male hormone testosterone.

Voracity, severe dieting, excessive exercise, lack of sleep, lack of exercise, excessive eating of processed foods, and excessive use of hand sanitizer can damage the secretion of hormones and the function of hormone receptors themselves, resulting in abnormalities in the body. Symptoms of hormonal imbalance include acne, weight gain, increased fatigue, excessive sweating, bags under the eyes, depression, sagging breasts, and hair loss.

Like this, the flow of hormones that are in charge of important functions in our body and the occlusion of teeth are deeply related. Occlusal incongruity is caused by excessive force on the skull, which distorts the cranial sutures and disrupts the normal flow of hormones.

In some cases, swallowing movements may adversely affect the skull. Everyone swallows twice a minute during the day and once a minute while sleeping. In the mouth, occlusal contact between the teeth occurs whenever swallowing is performed. Over a 24-hour period, 2,400 occlusal contacts are made, and a force of 3.5 pounds is applied for each swallowing exercise. Therefore, arithmetically, a total force of 3 tons is applied in 24 hours. When chewing food, 300~400 pounds are applied to the posterior teeth, and the more the malocclusion, the greater the occlusal force.

In an ideal centric relation, an occlusal force of about 12 kg/cm^2 acts. However, when premature contact or occlusal interference is severe, an occlusal force of 74~100 kg/cm^2 acts. While this force is applied during occlusion, it adversely affects the nervous and hormonal systems.

In the case of malocclusion, the balance of the masticatory muscles is broken, and the suture of the skull is deformed, resulting in distortion of the dural membrane. This can distort the spine and affect the flow of hormones, the nervous system and cerebrospinal fluid, which can adversely affect the healt of the whole body. Therefore, an ideal good occlusion plays a crucial role in the balanced movement of the skull.

Wearing a CBK splint promotes normalization of hormones and the nervous system, and it increases immunity. When the spine is upright, all immune cells (T cell, B cell, NK cell) can respond immediately. Twisting of the cervical vertebrae and pelvis caused by dental occlusion abnormalities along with bad posture causes the spine to bend. Therefore, proper posture and dental occlusion stabilization are essential conditions for the health of the whole body.

Clinically, if the suture of the skull is distorted due to the force of 6~10 times of the masticatory muscles due to premature contact or occlusal interference, recovery of occlusion with prosthesis or a CBK Splint is effective to greatly reduce migraine, rhinitis, tinnitus, etc. I am seeing improvement in these symptoms.

05 Five Components of Whole-body Health

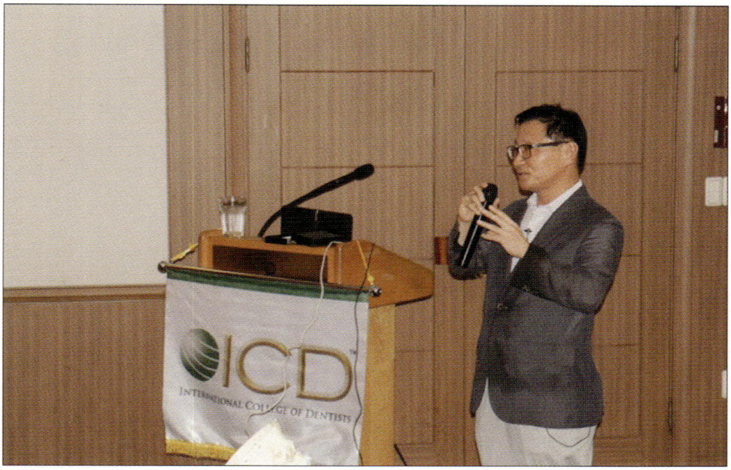

▲ Fig 82. Dr. Byungkee Choi lecturing at the International College of Dentists (ICD) Korean Conference

At the 16th International College of Prosthodontists (ICP) in 2015, I made a presentation on the five components of whole-body health in relation to CBK Splints. It was announced that the human body, such as the skull, spine, and pelvis, are organically connected as one, so posture, occlusion, and breathing have a mutual effect on the health of the whole body.

1 Stable dental occlusion

Maintaining ideal dental occlusion is very important for systemic health. Ordinary dental occlusion should be checked and corrected, and if occlusal disease is found, it should be treated without delay. If the dental occlusion is not correct and is distorted, the four masticatory muscles can be distorted by 6~10 times more than normal, causing distortion of the temporal bone and the second cervical vertebrae, which are the most important in the human body.

A person swallows about 2,400 times a day. In particular, swallowing movements that occur in an unconscious state during sleep can have a decisive effect on this distortion. At that time, occlusal diseases such as cervical abrasion, attrition, cracked teeth, and tooth mobility may be induced.

If there is occlusal disease, it can be identified using a T-scan and the teeth with occlusion problems can be adjusted to the ideal occlusion. If this is not satisfactory, a CBK Splint made with a 1.5 ㎜ metal strip bite should be worn during sleep and exercise. In this way, the inferior belly of the medial pterygoid muscle is completely relaxed, ultimately balancing the upper and lower jaws, thereby minimizing the effects on the skull caused by muscle distortion.

2 Straighten the spine

Gerald. H. Smith announced that diseases are induced in the human body as the skull, temporomandibular joint, pelvis, muscles, organs, nutritional status, and mental problems mutually and organically affect each other. All organs are connected to each of the 24 vertebrae, and if the posture is incorrect, the function of all organs decreases by 20~30 %. In the 1900's D.D. Palmer also famously said, "When the spine is standing upright, the Innate Intelligence (the immune system) works."

Bone can't beat muscle. Keep your back straight and open your chest. Also, walking properly is important for straightening the spine. The spine is the key that holds our body upright. Whole-body health can be maintained when the skull, spine, and pelvis are connected and organically function together. Therefore, building the spine correctly is to build good health.

Exercise is the most effective way to correct bad posture and maintain good posture. I was always tired and in poor physical condition 20 years ago until an acquaintance introduced me to a traditional martial art called 'Kicheonmun.' On the first day of this exercise, after an hour of back stretching exercises such as 'Danbaegong' and 'Yukhap,' all tiredness disappeared. Since then, I have never bent my back in treatment or in daily life, and I teach this to all my patients.

3 Abdominal breathing (Stress Control)

I learned a traditional martial art called 'Kicheonmun' 20 years ago, and I think it's the best exercise I've ever chosen. I am educating all patients to change chest breathing, which has become a daily habit, to abdominal breathing. Abdominal breathing, inhaling through the nose, is a gift created by God so that only humans can control the autonomic nervous system.

Modern people who live in a complex social structure suffer from various unavoidable stresses. Stress makes our mind and body hard, lowers our immunity, and causes various diseases. One of the ways to manage and relieve this stress is abdominal breathing.

In 1952, Buteyko, a Russian doctor, stated that diaphragmatic breathing, breathing through the nose, was more important than breathing through the mouth. The belly buttons on all newly born infants move up and down as they breathe. Adults normally breathe through their chest, but when climbing a mountain, they spontaneously breathe through their stomach. One of the reasons mountain climbing is good for health is the abdominal breathing that it causes.

When breathing, oxygen and carbon dioxide are exchanged in the lung cells. When inhaled, oxygen is absorbed and combined with nutrients from food to create energy. Waste products such as carbon dioxide that bodies does not need are expelled when people exhale. The breathing method is very important because a person must breathe without stopping for a moment while surviving. Abdominal breathing is the best breathing method for our body.

When practicing abdominal breathing for the first time, it is effective to practice lying down. The point of abdominal breathing is to relax your entire body and breathe slowly and deeply while being aware of the movement of your diaphragm. First, relax the muscles of the whole body, lie comfortably on the floor and close your eyes. Place one hand on your stomach and the other on your chest, so you can feel the muscle movement as you breathe. Inhale slowly and deeply through your nose for 2~4 seconds, placing your hand on your stomach and feeling it expand while you keep your shoulders and chest still. Hold your breath for 2~4 seconds after inhaling as much as you can. When exhaling, purse your lips and exhale as slowly as possible for about 4~8 seconds, making a whistling sound as you exhale. The time ratio of inhalation and exhalation is about 1:2, and in the beginning stage, it should be about 10 times a minute. As you get used to it, slow down to about 6~8 times a minute.

After learning how to breathe while lying down, you will be able to do it while sitting on a chair, standing, or walking slowly whenever you have time. The effect of abdominal breathing is to improve cardiorespiratory function, increase lung capacity, and increase oxygen and carbon dioxide exchange. When abdominal breathing moves the diaphragm, the vagus nerve attached to the diaphragm stimulates the parasympathetic nerve, helping to reduce insomnia, stress headaches, and anxiety disorders. In addition, when the parasympathetic nerve is activated, the mind becomes clear and concentration increases. In fact, if you measure your brain waves after doing abdominal breathing, you will see that alpha-waves, which appear when your mind is comfortable and your concentration is high, are activated. In addition, energy consumption increases during abdominal breathing, which has a diet effect, improves blood lipid status, and reduces cardiovascular disease.

When you are stressed, changes also occur in your mouth. When you are psychologically tense or anxious, your muscles harden due to the secretion of hormones, and the amount of saliva secretion also decreases, being reduced by up to 80 % in severe cases. When the secretion of saliva is reduced, the self-purification function in the oral cavity is weakened and bacterial activity increases. When this happens, teeth loosen, there is gingiva swelling, bleeding, pain, etc., and periodontal disease increases.

When you are stressed, your immunity decreases, and your resistance weakens. In addition, if there is a lot of stress, smoking or snacking increases, the oral condition becomes unclean, and plaque proliferates. When under a lot of stress, you may grind your teeth or clench them habitually when you go to bed. Bruxism or tooth clenching causes cervical abrasion, in which the boundary between teeth and the gingiva is broken by a force of 150~200 kg acting on the teeth. In particular, if there is occlusal interference because the upper and lower teeth do not fit well, stress can become severe and cause various dental diseases and chronic headaches. People with poor occlusion or occlusal interference complain of pain or sound in their temporomandibular joint area in front of the ear, and temporomandibular joint disease (trismus) that prevents them from opening their mouths fully. Stress is the main cause of three major dental diseases: tooth decay, periodontal disease, and temporomandibular joint disease.

It is important to be mentally stable through abdominal breathing and meditation, exercise appropriately, live with a pleasant mind, and relieve stress through hobbies with positive thinking and a relaxed mind.

4 Meditation(Mind Control)

Meditation is a mental process in which practitioners calmly close their eyes and concentrate on one place to clear their thoughts and promote relaxation of the mind and body. Meditation is directing the mind to realize one's true self. So, in various religions, it has been developed as a way to train the mind, such as Zen or meditative prayer. It is widely used as a health method by modern people who are under a lot of stress to manage their stress and find peace of mind and body. People do what they think. Therefore, it is necessary to reduce thoughts of the past and future and focus only on the present. I focus only on breathing while doing abdominal breathing, and I also use the method taught in the Lotus Sutra, such as 'Thank you.'

Meditation requires a considerable amount of training, but it can also be done as a daily way to calm the body and lighten the mind. First, you need to find a time and place to meditate. I like a quiet place where my concentration will not be disturbed. Listening to quiet music or using aromatherapy to block out noise can also help. When you are ready, take the most comfortable position. Meditation can be done lying down, sitting, or walking. Breathing is important in meditation, and abdominal breathing is essential. Take slow, deep breaths, focus your mind, and find one element to focus on. Select a specific object, a certain recitation, or an image and focus on that target. It is also good to create and memorize prayers from your own religion or belief.

This kind of meditation is effective when you enjoy it on your own as you get used to it through training for a considerable period of time. Meditation can be used as a method of mind control. Scientific studies have also shown that meditation has a positive effect on the autonomic nervous system and the flow of hormones, thereby providing psychological stability and relieving stress, thereby contributing to overall health.

* Have a quiet time for about 15 minutes before starting anything!
* Make it a habit to not start anything until your mind is calm!
* Seek God's help for a fresh start every day!

5 Environment (Diet and Exercise)

Modern people who love themselves try to do well in exercise and eating. In the past, malnutrition was a problem, but now overnutrition and contaminated food cause many diseases.

When choosing food, choose fresh food that is not contaminated with pesticides or chemicals. Natural foods such as brown rice and whole grains are better than processed and refined ones. Beware of powdered foods and oxidized fats. It is important to avoid unbalanced or overeating by planning your diet so that your body gets the nutrients it needs in a balanced way.

It is important to ensure that each part of our body functions smoothly through proper exercise. Exercise should be selected according to one's physical strength and health condition. Choose an exercise that you can do consistently every day, and balance aerobic exercise, such as running, with anaerobic exercise, such as strength training. Sports that can be enjoyed with family or friends are also desirable. The most common and recommended exercise is light running or fast walking.

References

- Kim Jae-gon (2019), The dental story of children and adolescents told by experts (Korean Academy of Pediatric Dentistry Promotional Booklet). Seoul: Sewon Cultural Publishing Co.
- Lee Sang-bok (2019), Dental Health 365 (Seoul Metropolitan Dental Association Public Relations Booklet), Seoul: Arab Edit
- Lee Youngjun(2019), Jaw joint balance therapy, Seoul: Fish Forest
- Co-authored by Choi Dae-gyun and Lee Seong-bok and 22 others (1997), Occlusal terms and illustrations, Seoul: The Korean Maxillofacial Occlusal Society.
- Imai Toshihiro, Imai Mayumi, translating by Sewon Jang (2010), Clinical occlusion Prosthetic Treatment, Seoul: Quintessence Korea
- Gerald H. Smith, B.S.D.D.S. (1983), CRANIAL DENTAL SACRAL COMPLEX, American and Canadian Dentist Manual, Seoul: Daehannarae Publishing House.
- Perter E. Dawson, DDS / John C. Cranham, DDS, Translating by Kim Seong-hoon · Jeong Ki-won (2019), Dawson's Complete USA, MOSBY ELSEVIER, ISBN-13
- Peter E. Dawson (2012), Functional Occlusion From TMJ to Smile Design, Philadelphia, PA, USA, Mosby Elsevier, ISBN-13

Reference Thesis

- Belser UC, Hannam AG. The contribution of the deep fibers of the masseter muscle to selected tooth -clenching and chewing tasks. J Prosthet Dent 1986:56:629-635.
- Burgett FG, Ramfjord SP, Nissle RR, Morrison EC, Charbeneau TD, Caffesse RG. A randomized trial of occlusal adjustment in the treatment of periodontitis patients. J Clin Periodontol. 1992; 19:381-387.
- Hallmon WW. Occlusal trauma: Effect and impact on the periodontium. Consensus report: Occlusal trauma. American Academy of Periodontology, 1999 International Workshop for a Classification of Periodontal Diseases and Conditions. Annals of Periodontalogy 1999;1:102-108.
- Grickman I, Smulow JB. Alterations in the pathway of gingival inflammation into the underlying tissues induced by excessive occlusal force. J Periodontol 1962:33:7-13.
- Hallmon WW, Harrel SK. Occlusal analysis, diagnosis and management in the practice of periodontics. J Periodontol 2000 2004;34:151-164.
- Harrel SK, Nunn ME. The effect of occlusal discrepancies on periodontitis. II. Relationship of occlusal treatment to the progression of periodontal disease. J Periodontol 2001;72:495-505.
- Harrel SK. Occlusal forces as a risk factor for periodontal disease. Periodontology 2000, J Periodontol 2000, 2003;32:111-117.
- Harrel SK, Nunn ME. The association of occlusal contacts with the presence ofincreased periodontal probing depth. J Clin Periodontol. 2009 Dec;36(12):1035-1042.
- Lindhe J, Ericsson 1. The effect of elimination of jiggling forces on periodontally exposed teeth in the dog. J Periodontol 1982; 53: 562-567
- Lindhe J, Ericsson I. Influence of trauma from occlusion on reduced but healthy periodontal tissues in dogs. J Clin Periodontol 1976; 3: 110-22.

- Lindhe J, Svanberg G. Influence of trauma from occlusion on progression of experimental periodontitis in the beagle dog. J Clin Periodontol 1974;13-14
- Manns A. Influence of group function and canine guidance on electromyographic activity of elevator muscles. J Prosthet Dent 1987:57(4): 494-501.
- Meitner S. Co-destructive factors of marginal periodontitis and repetitive mechanical injury. J Dent Res 1975:54 Spec no C:C78-85.
- Polson AM. Interrelationship of inflammation and tooth mobility (trauma) in pathogenesis of periodontal disease. J Clin Periodontol 1980;7:351-360.
- Polson AM. Trauma and progression of marginal periodontitis in squirrel monkeys. II. Co-destructive factors of periodontitis and mechanically-produced injury. J Periodontal Res 1974:9.108-113.
- Posselt U. Studies in the mobility of the human mandible. Acta Odont. Scand. 10, Suppl. 10:19, 1952.
- Proye M, Caton J, Polson A. Initial healing of periodontal pockets after a single episode of root planing monitored by controlled probing forces. J Periodontol 1982:53:296-301.
- Stillman PR (1917) The management of pyorrhea. Stillman PR (1926) What is traumatic occlusion and how can it be diagnosed and corrected.
- Waerhaug J. The angular bone defect and its relationship to trauma from occlusion and downgrowth of subgingival plaque. J Clin Periodontol 1979:6:61-82.
- Waerhaug J. The infrabony Pocket and its Relationship to Trauma from Occlusion and Subgingival Plague. J Periodontol, 1979; 50:355-365.
- O Weinman J. Progress of gingival inflammation into the supporting structure of the teeth. J Periodontol 1941:12:71-76

■ CBK Splint Q & A

Q1. What is the difference between conventional splints and the CBK Splint?

First, it is installed after an ideal occlusion has been achieved using a T-scan.

That is, the occlusal time of the teeth is adjusted to within 0.3 seconds, and the disclusion time is adjusted to within 0.4 seconds. If possible, try to match the centric relation and maximal intercuspal position. As a result, the inferior belly of the lateral pterygoid muscle is relaxed, and the distortion of the cranial suture is released, which affects the balance of hormones and the nervous system.

Second, a 1.5 mm metal strip bite, an invention for which the author obtained a patent, is used to obtain the centric relation.

Third, the CBK Splint was produced to improve the whole-body health.

In the past, splints were installed for the treatment of temporomandibular joints, but CBK Splints help improve whole-body health by combining correct posture, exercise, abdominal breathing, meditation, with proper eating habits.

Q 2. Do CBK Splints come with any side effects?

Wearing a CBK Splint is a bit inconvenient at first, but there is almost no discomfort if the centric relation and the maximal intercuspal position has been adjusted once or twice before they are worn. Existing soft splints can have a good effect temporarily, but there are problems with long-term use due to distorted temporomandibular joints and deformed teeth, so care must be taken when using them.

Q 3. How would you briefly explain the whole-body health benefits of CBK Splints?

When a CBK Splint is installed, the atlas and axis vertebrae acquire ideal positions and shapes. Then, the muscles connected to the atlas and the axis vertebrae relax, the spine stands upright, and the masticatory muscles move above the center, and the inferior belly of the lateral pterygoid muscle relaxes. This stabilizes the skull, affects hormones and the nervous system, and facilitates the flow of cerebrospinal fluid.

I am continuing to study the correlation between CBK Splints and whole-body health through scientific methods such as clinical experience and questionnaires.

Q4. Should I wear a CBK Splint only when I sleep at night?

Wearing it while sleeping is the most important thing. When swallowing (saliva swallowing) in an unconscious state at bedtime, there is 6~10 times more force than normal. This force causes distortion of the masticatory muscles and affects the distortion of the most important temporal bone and second cervical vertebrae (axis) in the human body. At this time, occlusal diseases such as cervical abrasion, attrition, cracked teeth, and tooth mobility may also be induced.

If the CBK Splint is matched from the centric relation to the maximal intercuspal position and is ideally adjusted, you can wear it while exercising or during the day.

Q5. What is the most uncomfortable thing about wearing a CBK Splint?

It may be a bit uncomfortable for 3 weeks when first wearing it, but after it has been adjusted one or two times, the discomfort disappears. However, do not try putting it on when you actually go to bed, rather put the CBK Splint on immediately after brushing your teeth after dinner and then go to sleep sometime later.

Q 6. What are the advantages of the patented metal strip bite?

It is easier to achieve a centric relation with my patented metal strip bite than when with the traditional method that uses paraffin wax. Because I adjust the occlusion with a metal strip bite, this minimizes the need for adjustment after splint fabrication

Q 7. How do you adjust the CBK Splint?

At first, using 80μm horseshoe-shaped articulating paper, adjust so that a line is formed in the anterior area and there is one dot in the posterior area. Then, 3 days and 1 week later, readjust it with finer articulating paper and check it every 3 months.

Q 8. How long will I have to wear the CBK Splint?

Conventional splints are used only when there is temporomandibular joint disease or when there is pain.

Since the CBK Splint is worn to improve the whole-body health, we recommend that you use it for the rest of your life. After wearing a CBK Splint, periodontal disease is significantly reduced, and deep sleep is achieved. In addition, rhinitis, tinnitus, etc. are reduced, and good results such as improvement of nasolabial folds are being seen. A word of advice: the splint should be disinfected with denture cleaner about twice a week.

Q 9. Can patients with partial dentures or implant use it?

In most cases, patients with periodontal disease or implants have poor occlusion no matter how well they brush their teeth. In this case, tooth clenching or bruxism at bedtime can easily cause cervical abrasion, attrition, cracked teeth, periodontal disease, etc. Therefore, occlusal adjustment and a CBK Splint are essential for patients with periodontal disease or implants.

In addition, it is important for patients with partial dentures to remove them and insert a CBK Splint to minimize bite force while sleeping.

Q 10. Is there any evidence that stretching the spine, abdominal breathing, and wearing splints improves whole-body health?

Palmer and Tinbergen announced that a correct spinal posture affects the health of the whole body. Until the 1980s, many scholars, such as Smith and Fonder, also conducted whole-body health studies to determine the effects of spine, occlusion, and temporomandibular joint distortion on hormones and the nervous system.

More recently, Kirstein announced that there is 6~10 times greater distortion of the masticatory muscles due to premature contact or occlusal interference than with a good occlusion. After announcing the CBK Splint effects based on the scholarly theories, the author can confirm good results in more than 5,000 cases.

In the future, we plan to contribute to the further improvement of the health of more people by expanding the application of CBK Splints through combined research with specialists in many other fields such as internal medicine, otolaryngology, neurology, orthopedics, and oriental medicine.

Q 11. How should we manage CBK Splint?

When wiping the splint in the morning after wearing it, clean the inside with a toothbrush while holding it under cold running water.

- ○ It typically takes 2~3 weeks to adapt to wearing a splint. After an adaptation period and wearing the device for a long time, fine adjustment of the teeth and device is required due to changes in the temporomandibular joint disc.
- ○ After installation, disinfect the splint with denture cleaner about twice a week. Add some denture cleaner to water and soak the splint for about 5 minutes, then rinse it with clean water before use.
- ○ When not in use, wipe clean and store in a container with water or without water.
- ○ Visit the dentist once every 3 months to check for changes in the dentition and device, and make sure you have a healthy mouth.
- ○ Try to have a positive mind and wear the splint while sleeping, but do not bite it.
- ○ If you feel uncomfortable in the morning after wearing the device, go to the dentist and have it adjusted to make it more comfortable.
- ○ Always straighten your back, keep the right posture, and walk with the right posture.

■ Experience with a CBK Splint Review

■ **Kim Oh-soo (former Prosecutor General. Current chair professor at Chonnam National University)**

-Thinking of the late Director Byungkee Choi -

On July 6, 2023, I received a strange phone call. Like all of us, I frequently get advertisement and survey calls so I often ignore my phone. On this particular day, the phone number looked familiar and there seemed to be an urgency to it, so I checked and discovered it was Director Choi's hospital phone number.

In 2016, while serving as the chief prosecutor of the Seoul Northern District Prosecutor's Office, I first became aware of the director who volunteered for legal affairs and prosecution. Coincidentally, when I said that I was suffering from a sick wisdom tooth, he asked me to come to the hospital and we got to know each other as doctor and patient. After more than 20 years of living in the difficult role of prosecutor, it seemed that my teeth were in bad shape! Drinking, smoking, and stress at work may have been the cause. My wisdom tooth extraction was postponed until the damaged gingiva and teeth were treated first. One day after a dental treatment, the director introduced me to the CBK Splint and suggested that I try it. I immediately agreed because my dental treatment with this doctor had gone well and trusted him. I have been using the CBK Splint since the summer of 2016 until now, about 7 years later. I put it on my lower teeth before bed. It is a bit cumbersome because the splint has to be soaked in water during the day and occasionally, I have to disinfect it with denture cleaner. In addition, when I travel, I have to pay attention to how I store it.

After 7 years, the Splint has become a natural part of me. With it, I feel like I'm getting a good night's sleep, and it seems to be helping to keep my teeth strong. I think it is a great benefit to my health, perhaps because I sleep well, and my teeth are properly cared for. I think it has the effect of preventing my teeth from excessive wear or damage due to grinding teeth while I sleep.

I was shocked to hear the news of the death of Director Choi, who was always energetic and healthy. However, I am sorry that I was unable to attend the funeral because I was traveling to Cheongsando with my acquaintances, and my heart is heavy. I still wear my CBK Splint made by the director every day when I sleep. Whenever I wear it, I think of Director Choi. He always made the hospital lively by calling out the names and positions of patients, doctors, and hygienists with a strong and positive voice.

I will continue to wear and live with my CBK Splint made by the director. As I do, I will think of Director Choi. I hope Director Choi Byungkee, who smiled widely while he was in the world, is resting in peace. (July 7, 2023)

■ Pastor Ilhwa Lee

As a result of wearing a CBK Splint, I obtained the following:

1. History of tooth and periodontal disease

Since 1999, I have had a habit of sleeping with my molars clenched every night due to stress from work. At the time, the gingiva around my right molar and second tooth was so inflamed and decayed that I had no choice but to undergo surgery for periodontal disease. This happened around the year 2000. Soon afterwards, my upper left wisdom tooth was on the verge of being completely cracked because the innermost molar on the upper left side of the molar cracked vertically, and the second tooth next to the molar was also cracked. Initially, I had it treated with a prosthetic, and I've been maintaining it until now.

Unfortunately, due to frequent stress from my job, my lower right molar began to crack again, and the lower right molar also cracked, and even my periodontal disease was in a dangerous state. This tooth has also been maintained until now by reinforcing the lower part of the tooth with a prosthesis and covering the cracked tooth. This was my periodontal situation more than a decade ago. In the meantime, the tooth right next to my right molar was cracked, so I had no choice but to replace it with a prosthesis.

Between about 2000 and during the next 5~6 years, I was in pain due to my teeth caused by my habit of sleeping with my teeth tightly clenched due to job stress. When I talked about my cracked teeth to other hospitals, the other hospitals wanted to extract the teeth and replace them with implants.

This didn’t seem right because the cracked tooth was well attached and had a prosthetic cover, so I was able to use it for about 20 years since then.

2. History and effect of wearing a Sprint

Knowing that I sleep with my teeth clenched due to the stress of work, the director recommended a CBK Splint for me. My teeth haven’t cracked since I started wearing the CBK Splint, and I have been able to get a good night's sleep.

Effect 1) The risk and worry of cracked teeth has been eliminated.

My job was highly stressful. However, when I went to bed wearing the CBK Splint, even if I had to bite my molars tightly, the lifting force of the upper teeth was stably and evenly distributed to the lower teeth, so not much strain was putt on any one tooth such as my molars.

Effect 2) The phenomenon of my lower teeth shifting toward the center was eliminated in spite of dental aging.

One of the phenomena that occurs as teeth age is that the lower teeth gradually move from both molars to the center of the lower teeth, causing the lower center teeth to become crooked. However, after wearing my CBK Splint, this tendency to lean went away.

For reference, I wear a CBK Splint on my lower teeth, but my wife wears a CBK Splint on her upper teeth which doesn't reduce the centering of the lower teeth. I think it seems to be more effective to wear a CBK Splint on the lower teeth.

Effect 3) Wearing the sprint expands the oral space, making it easier to breathe.

Effect 4) There is psychological stability.

After wearing the CBK Splint, there was a sense of psychological stability that didn't put too much pressure on it, so I got a good night's sleep because I felt feel comfortable.

Effect 5) Even if I wasn't able to wear the splint every day, wearing it only a couple of times a week seemed to help my sleep.

After chewing tough meat or vegetables, I could feel the roots of my molars stinging my gingiva. By wearing a CBK Splint while I slept, it felt like my molars were back in place. Especially if I ate foods such as tough meat and sashimi, my molars got overcrowded. By wearing a CBK Splint to bed, the next morning I could clearly feel that my teeth were back in place.

If you wear a CBK Splint when you sleep, you can feel that the space in your mouth has expanded, and you can breathe naturally, so you can sleep well. Rhinitis symptoms also feel better.

Something to consider, if you catch a cold, you need to be sure to disinfect your Splint at this time, as nasal mucus is passed into the airway without mixing with saliva, which can cause a sore throat. But on the other hand, wearing a CBK Splint makes it much easier to breathe.

■ 14th Korea Coast Guard Commissioner Hong Ik-tae

I am Hong Ik-tae, the 14th Commissioner of the Korea Coast Guard. I still can't believe that Director Choi Byungkee has passed away. I suddenly remember.

For over 20 years, not just me but also my wife and three daughters have been going to the Director Choi. I am eternally thankful for my good health due to Director Choi's meticulous dental care.

It’s good to see you passionately researching and disseminating CBK Splints so that everyone can live a healthy life as well as good dental health. You continue to develop the splint and are working to the point of losing your health to bring it to the world. When you wake up in the morning after using a CBK Splint, your gingiva is tight. Even though I am in my mid to late 60s, I feel that my teeth are not deteriorating but are actually getting healthier. One of my daughters complained that she had headaches because she couldn't get a good night's sleep. All three daughters are using splints now, and their dental health as well as their skin and posture have improved. I think all of this is the result of Dr. Choi's research, and I am grateful again. I hope that your son, Director Choi Youngkyun, will follow his father's footsteps and try to help everyone live a healthy life through splint research and distribution.

Thank you!

■ Kim Hwa-ja (former Employment and Labor Minister Lee Ki-kwon's family)

I went to sleep with a CBK Splint upon the recommendation of Director Choi Byungkee. I had a habit of grinding my teeth as I slept, so I always had a sore tooth in the morning. All this has disappeared.

■ Min kyung-gu (Anyang-dong, Manan-gu, Anyang City)

I have bad teeth, so I am have gotten 10 implants and it's been 10 years since they were placed. Even so, I neglected dental care, so I often felt like my teeth were getting worse.

Since then, I have been using the CBK Splint that Dentist Choi Byungkee recommended. As a result, my teeth have felt comfortable and refreshed. And by wearing a CBK Splint every night, I have felt that not only my teeth were getting better, but also my health.

Then, two years ago, I went on a long-term overseas trip. I was very uncomfortable and anxious because I forgot to take my splint with me. When I was wearing my CBK Splint every night, I would wake up in the morning feeling refreshed and my teeth were held tightly, but after traveling without my CBK Splint, I felt like my teeth were shaking, food got caught between them, and my teeth didn't seem fit, so it made me feel anxious.

I found my CBK Splint right after I got home. As expected, when I tried to wear it, my teeth were deformed, and the splint didn't fit. This experience has convinced me that a CBK Splint will keep the inner teeth in their youthful shape. As soon as possible, I visited the dentist. After correction, I am again using splint and am very comfortable.

■ Park Dong-min (Executive Director, Korea Chamber of Commerce and Industry)

I usually do not go to hospitals or pharmacies when I get sick. Due to the nature of my work, I drank alcohol and smoked excessively, but was overconfident because I was innately healthy to some extent, but I had treated my body harshly repeatedly for over 30 years. Eventually, I developed serious problems with my gingiva and teeth.

At the persistent recommendation of an acquaintance, President

Jeong Ki-ok, I visited Director Choi Byungkee, who recently passed away. As a result of a CT exam, Director Choi found that my gingiva was not the problem, but rather I had a severe vascular disease with a high possibility of diabetes. In addition, I had almost no upper right jawbone, and the membrane that should have been between my mouth and eyes had melted and disappeared. Dental treatment was not possible in this condition, so Director Choi told me to get implants after first receiving internal medicine and otolaryngology treatment.

The next morning, after getting the rather shocking results from an internal medicine clinic near my house that I had a fasting blood sugar level of 250 and glycated hemoglobin of 12.3 at a university hospital, I told Dr. Choi that I should be able to start dental treatment in at about three months.

Over the course of a year, I received treatment while minimizing my drinking and smoking, and I had a total of 11 implants placed. Now, I am more satisfied with my teeth than I was with the teeth my parents gave me, and I feel apologetic to my parents.

At the time, I vividly recall Director Choi saying, "The reason Park's implants need to be completed quickly is not because of his teeth, but because he needs to be in a state where he can wear a splint."

After that, I did not forget to wear my CBK Splints every night. After a few months, I started hearing people around me saying that my face was getting younger and younger. Of course, as my face got younger, my physical strength improved. Specifically, my sinusitis, which was a chronic disease, mysteriously disappeared, so I am eternally grateful to Director Choi.

Director Choi's dedication to patients, his passion for developing treatment technology, and his volunteer work among the socially underprivileged, and especially the amazing effects of his CBK Splint leave a great legacy.

Director Choi Byungkee now lives in heaven, I am eternally grateful to him. Rest in peace.

■ Kang Cheol-yong (Chief of Medical Asia Steering Committee)
<CBK Splint protecting teeth from gingiva inflammation>

When I turned 50, I had two gingiva surgeries due to continued inflammation of my upper molars. By the time I was in my mid-50s, my periodontitis had become chronic, so I ended up having to have my teeth removed and implants placed in their place. Three years later, I also lost two of my upper and lower molars for the same reason and had needed implants.

At the time, Dr. Choi Byungkee said that my lower jaw was strong, so I was putting a burden on my teeth while I slept, which caused inflammation and poor quality of sleep. Director Choi, while giving me implants, said I must wear a CBK Splint to prevent tooth loss in the future and to maintain my current condition. He said there was no other way.

At that time, I bought a CBK Splint at Director Choi's recommendation, but the effect was doubtful. Consequently, I was repeatedly started and stopped wearing the CBK Splint.

Director Choi could tell that I was doing this so he told me that I have a habit of clenching my teeth while I sleep, so there is a limit what can be done for my dental inflammation with surgery alone, and again asked me to wear the sprint consistently.

Because of Director Choi's affectionate recommendation, I started wearing the splint every day without skipping exception. Not only did the tooth inflammation disappear, but various changes appeared in my body.

First, I had a habit of clenching my teeth while I slept, so my teeth were getting worse, but after wearing the CBK Splint, the symptoms of abrasion and hypersensitivity disappeared.

Also, before wearing the splint, my body felt heavy when I awoke and my fatigue did not go away, but about a month after starting to wear the CBK Splint consistently, I was able to sleep more deeply, and I could feel my body getting lighter in the morning.

So far, I've been wearing a splint consistently for about 3 years. Other molars that used to be inflamed didn't need to be extracted after wearing the CBK Splint and are still well maintained.

Now, my CBK Splint has become a "must-have" tool for me when I sleep. Even when I travel or go on a business trip, it's the first thing I take with me in my toiletries.

The CBK Splint is a great invention that helps with dental problems which cannot be treated with surgery or medicine. I would like to share with many people that that CBK Splints which look like a mouthpiece have a big impact on dental and mental health.

■ Lim Heung-soon (male. Professor, Hanyang Cyber University, former Director General of KBS)

It was in 2016 when Director Choi Byungkee recommended that I get fitted for a splint. I ordered the splint but was dubious about its benefits. I really didn't expect it to work all that well. Even so, in the hopes that it might work, I tried wearing it to bed.

The first few days were quite uncomfortable because I was not used to it. After the first few nights of trying to wear it, I would wake up in the morning and find the splint rolling under my feet, but after 4 or 5 days, my resistance to wearing it gradually disappeared.

After about a week of actually using it, the effects gradually started to show. When I was tired, I would snore, but that decreased remarkably as I wore the splint. My wife told me that not only did I snore less, but the severity of my snoring had decreased.

I also had the habit of grinding my teeth when I was especially tired. There were times I would wake up in surprise because I had been grinding my teeth while I slept. Thankfully, after using the splint, this habit has improved quite a bit. I heard that some people bite their teeth with strong force unknowingly while sleeping, which damages their teeth and adversely affects the brain. Fortunately, wearing a splint seems to have the effect of mitigating this phenomenon.

My breathing while sleeping has also improved a lot. In the past, my throat would be dry when I awoke after sleeping with my mouth open. Sometimes this gave me a sore throat and cough. However, after using the splint, I naturally breathe through my nose, and the quality of my sleep has improved.

Director Choi Byungkee, who is now deceased, used to emphasize whenever I saw him for medical treatment, that I must wear my CBK Splint at night, saying, "If you wear a splint, your life will change." I don't know if my life has changed, but it seems to be a clear fact that when I sleep, my jaw strength is relieved and I breathe through my nose instead of my mouth, which contributes to my health.